Leading Your Healthcare Organization Through a Merger or Acquisition

Your board, staff, or clients may also benefit from this book's insight. For more information on quantity discounts, contact the Health Administration Press Marketing Manager at (312) 424-9470.

This publication is intended to provide accurate and authoritative information in regard to the subject matter covered. It is sold, or otherwise provided, with the understanding that the publisher is not engaged in rendering professional services. If professional advice or other expert assistance is required, the services of a competent professional should be sought.

Reprinted April 2015

Library of Congress Cataloging-in-Publication Data

Leading your healthcare organization through a merger or acquisition /Alan Zuckerman, editor.
    p. cm.
Includes bibliographical references.
ISBN 978-1-56793-360-4 (alk. paper)
1. Medical corporations--Mergers. I. Zuckerman, Alan M.
  R728.2.L43 2010
  610.68--dc22

                2010030746

The paper used in this publication meets the minimum requirements of American National Standard for Information Sciences—Permanence of Paper for Printed Library Materials, ANSI Z39.48-1984. ∞™

Acquisitions editor: Janet Davis; Project manager: Jennifer Seibert; Cover designer: Marisa Jackson; Layout: BookComp

Found an error or a typo? We want to know! Please e-mail it to hap1@ache.org, and put "Book Error" in the subject line.

For photocopying and copyright information, please contact Copyright Clearance Center at www.copyright.com or at (978) 750-8400.

Health Administration Press
A division of the Foundation of the American
    College of Healthcare Executives
One North Franklin Street, Suite 1700
Chicago, IL 60606-3529
(312) 424-2800

Foreword

Mergers and acquisitions are strategic options that many healthcare leaders consider in response to changing economic conditions. Whether facing economic difficulties and uncertainties, capital needs that are outstripping capital access and availability, growing quality and safety imperatives that require scale to address, or other environmental changes and challenges, providers of all types are thinking about forming new relationships with others. As we enter another period of strategic repositioning in response to recently enacted healthcare reform legislation, *Leading Your Healthcare Organization Through a Merger or Acquisition* is a timely resource for executives and board members who need to understand the broad and complex topics related to mergers and acquisitions.

Our experience in developing BJC HealthCare, one of the largest not-for-profit systems in the United States, is that, although each transaction is different, all involve common concerns. These common concerns, especially in the delicate, early stages of discussion and negotiation, are the primary subjects of this book:

- **Vision**: What can we accomplish together that we could not accomplish independently?
- **Culture**: Can differences in values and organizational behaviors be bridged if we come together?
- **Governance**: Can we balance the parties' egos, desire for control, history, style, personalities, structure, and finances to fashion an overall design, approach, and team?
- **Organization and operations**: Can we create organizational and operational structures that serve the parties effectively and efficiently?
- **Physician impacts and politics**: Can we show benefit to physicians and navigate often difficult personal concerns?

- **Clinical/quality impacts**: Can we grow and improve clinical programs and enhance quality and safety better as partners?
- **Financial benefits**: Can we reduce costs, increase revenue, and improve overall financial performance and position?
- **Other issues and concerns**: Can we address human resources, legal/regulatory, religious, and other threshold challenges?

If you're a leader in an organization strategically considering being a market consolidator, in a smaller organization thinking of joining forces with a larger one, in an area where two providers are competing for business and only 1.5 or fewer is needed, or in some other situation where consolidation with others might make sense, this book can help you get started evaluating and perhaps initiating a merger or an acquisition. It's a nuts and bolts guide to the first stage of planning for a merger or an acquisition and should help you get to stage two—actually crafting and carrying out the transaction.

This book addresses the big issues and concerns that emerge in almost every discussion about merger and acquisition. Keep these challenges (and strategies for how you're going to address them) front and center as you move forward. Resist the temptation to get buried in the weeds, and keep driving toward the larger goals you set at the outset. Don't underestimate how difficult it is to achieve meaningful change, and understand that what you're trying to do will require endurance of some short-term turbulence in exchange for long-term success. It is a journey that may very well take years. Good luck.

Steven H. Lipstein
President and CEO
BJC HealthCare
St. Louis, Missouri

What Could We Accomplish Together That We Cannot Do Alone?

MARIA FINARELLI

All proposed healthcare mergers and acquisitions stem from the rationale that, together, the merging organizations can be more successful and achieve a higher purpose than they could achieve on their own. This rationale considers the future competitiveness of one or both organizations and community needs and benefits.

Similar to the vision statement developed during strategic planning, the rationale describes a preferred future state that is ten or more years away. The future state is a stretch target that motivates, energizes, and inspires the combining organizations.

Guidelines to developing a vision for a merged organization are listed in Exhibit 1.1.

> **EXHIBIT 1.1: Guidelines to Developing a Vision for a Merged Organization**
>
> - Describes a purpose that can be achieved only collectively
> - Defines what success looks like ten or more years in the future
> - Considers the benefits that will accrue to the community and the potential partners as a result of the merger
> - Inspires and challenges the organization
> - Is briefly stated and clearly articulated

BENEFITS TO EACH ORGANIZATION

Organizations frequently cite the potential for growth as part of their rationale for joining together. In many cases, the merging organizations can develop new services or clinical capabilities because after unifying they have sufficient mass to support them and to attract new subspecialty physicians to the area. Merging organizations often establish a presence in one or more new geographic markets or solidify the market position of one or both organizations. The combined entity's capacity might also enable existing programs to be expanded or relocated.

Improved performance is often another expected outcome of a proposed merger or acquisition. The combining organizations typically aspire to provide a higher quality of care and better patient experiences. In response to the growing number of initiatives that link payment rates and clinical outcomes, merger rationales today place particular emphasis on quality of care. Other desired outcomes include shared best practices, including those related to clinical protocols and care processes, and the delivery of integrated, coordinated care.

Most potential merger partners anticipate that financial benefits will occur as a result of the new relationship. Organizations of all sizes identify opportunities to improve access to capital, attain financial security, and benefit from economies of scale. Financially stable organizations may view potential mergers or acquisitions as a way to increase operating margins, spread overhead across a larger base of operations, or achieve a certain scale or volume. The ability to fund facility improvements, new construction, investments in technology, and other growth initiatives is often paramount and will help meet the demand for services.

Spectrum Health, based in Grand Rapids, Michigan, continues its development as a fully integrated healthcare system. In early 2009, the system included seven hospitals and the Priority Health insurance company and employed nearly 100 doctors in the recently formed Spectrum Health Medical Group. Michigan Medical, P.C. (mmpc®) was the largest physician-owned, multispecialty physician group in West Michigan, with 200 doctors and 100 other healthcare providers in more than 30 specialties. The two organizations had engaged in talks off and on since 2006. The initial round of talks ended when several physicians objected to being excluded from the discussions, and in 2008, governance issues led mmpc to withdraw, following a decision that remaining a physician-owned practice was in the best interest of the community (Spectrum Health 2009; *Grand Rapids Press* 2009; Schroder 2008). Discussions resumed in the spring of 2009.

Expected benefits of a merger included the ability to provide more effective, accessible, coordinated care to the residents of Western Michigan and to control healthcare costs by minimizing duplication. The medical director of mmpc indicated that "doing business as usual is not an option for physicians. It makes more sense to be in a system that's not wasting resources." The merger, which was effective August 2009, formalized an existing alignment between the two organizations that had spanned several years and, for Spectrum, furthered the organization's goal to become a medical destination similar to Mayo Clinic and Cleveland Clinic (Spectrum Health 2009; *Grand Rapids Press* 2009).

The merger between Sun Health and Banner Health is another example that clearly illustrates the benefits two organizations can realize by joining together. In September 2007, Sun Health owned two hospitals and several other healthcare facilities in rapidly growing communities northwest of Phoenix, Arizona, but its efforts to meet the healthcare needs of area residents were placing a strain on its resources. Banner Health operated 16 hospitals in six western states, including eight in the Phoenix metropolitan area. As part of Banner's aggressive growth plans, significant expansion projects were under way at several facilities and two new hospitals were under construction. However, all but one of Banner's Arizona facilities were located in Phoenix and the cities of Mesa and Scottsdale to the east (Alltucker 2007; Gonzales 2007).

For Sun Health, a merger meant financial stability, access to new sources of capital, and more advanced technology. Banner would be able to solidify its market leadership position, expand its geographic reach, and establish a significant presence in growth markets without having to build new facilities. Shortly after the merger of the two systems was announced, Banner acquired Arizona Medical Clinic, a multispecialty group practice with nearly 90 physicians and 15 midlevel providers who already admitted all of their patients to Sun Health facilities (Gonzales 2007). The deal between Banner Health and Sun Health closed in September 2008 (Alltucker 2008).

ENHANCING COMPETITIVENESS

For most organizations evaluating a potential merger or acquisition,

a driving force is the prospect of implementing strategies that would not be feasible independently. These strategies may direct investments in facilities and/or new technology and the recruitment of new subspecialty expertise, but the majority of initiatives can be categorized as one of two kinds of growth opportunities: improved market position and clinical services development.

Increased market share and greater retention of patients who might otherwise choose to leave the area to obtain care are common elements of the rationale for two organizations in the same region to come together. With more critical mass and broader geographic coverage in the market, the combined entity will be better able to defend against competitive threats and initiatives. Another motivating factor might be to secure more physician referrals, particularly if several area physician groups have merged or if competing hospitals and systems have stepped up efforts to acquire practices. Some organizations may be driven by the prospect of improved negotiating leverage with private payers, although in many cases, the consolidation of the insurance industry over the last decade has made this factor less important.

The development of new services is also frequently mentioned in merger announcements or discussions. A larger service area population and patient base often justify building a regional center of excellence or subspecialty expertise. In other cases, consolidation of the merging organizations' programs might justify development of a new service. Alternatively, the increased patient volume resulting from the combination of two referral streams might be a reason to establish a new component along the continuum of care.

In April 2009, Johns Hopkins Health System and Suburban Hospital Healthcare System, two organizations that operated in separate but adjacent markets, announced an agreement to integrate. At the time, Johns Hopkins Health System, a member of Johns Hopkins Medicine, included two acute care hospitals in Baltimore, Maryland, and a third in Columbia, Maryland, a bedroom community of Baltimore and Washington, DC. However, Johns Hopkins Health System did not have a presence in the nation's capital or any of its close suburbs. Suburban was a community-based, not-for-profit health system in Bethesda, Maryland, just outside the northwestern

city limits of Washington, DC. Suburban had established multiple clinical partnerships with the National Institutes of Health (located across the street from the hospital) and Johns Hopkins Medicine during the previous 13 years (Suburban Hospital 2009a).

Suburban, a financially strong hospital highly regarded in the community, initiated the discussions between the two systems. The hospital's leaders believed that integrating with Johns Hopkins Health System, a strong organization with an international reputation for excellence, would augment its clinical services and open up more opportunities for innovation, research, and education. The combined organization would also provide new opportunities to serve patients along the continuum of care and deliver coordinated and efficient care (Suburban Hospital 2009b).

A stronger, expanded regional integrated healthcare network would position Johns Hopkins Medicine to assume an important role in managing health for Maryland's population—a role particularly important in an era of healthcare reform and constrained resources. The new Johns Hopkins Medicine would also establish a presence in the Washington,

DC, healthcare market. Suburban's board leadership expressed the belief that the affiliation "will be recognized by future generations as a turning point for transforming the healthcare delivery process for our local community and, more broadly, for the greater Washington, DC, region." The merger became official in July 2009 (Suburban Hospital 2009a).

TANGIBLE COMMUNITY BENEFITS

When organizations come together, one or both entities envision achieving a stronger competitive position and better clinical and operational performance, gaining financial stability and access to capital, and developing a greater breadth and/or depth of services. In addition, mergers or affiliations bring important benefits to the communities served, such as those described in the previous example regarding the Johns Hopkins–Suburban affiliation. Specifically, a greater breadth and depth of service offerings means patients have access to more healthcare options locally, reducing the need to travel longer distances for specialty and subspecialty care. Patients in the community will also benefit from better coordination and continuity of care.

Certain costs should be avoidable following a merger or affiliation because duplicative capital investments and program development initiatives that would have been made are no longer necessary. Selectively consolidating and strengthening clinical services will improve the quality of care and reduce costs. Additional cost reductions are typically realized once administrative and clinical support services are combined. While historically cost reductions have not translated into price reductions for consumers and payers, there is the likelihood that under healthcare reform, both government and private payers and consumers will begin to benefit from these cost reductions.

In many cases, successful mergers stimulate the local economy. Initiatives implemented by the combined entity may create jobs, either within the newly merged organization or in companies in related industries. Coordination of care for the vulnerable populations in the community should also improve following a merger or affiliation because the organizations can pool their resources.

The merger between Sanford Health and MeritCare demonstrates the effect that combining forces can have on the surrounding community. Sanford Health includes Sanford USD Medical Center and a network of community hospitals and clinics in South Dakota, southwest Minnesota, northwest Iowa, and northeast Nebraska. MeritCare, North Dakota's largest health system, has many regional sites in North Dakota and northwest Minnesota. Both systems are perceived to be leaders in their respective regions and are committed to system integration as the way to deliver quality, cost-effective care. The two organizations signed a letter of intent to merge in July 2009 and a definitive agreement in November 2009 (Sanford Health–MeritCare 2009a).

The unified efforts of Sanford Health and MeritCare are expected to create growth opportunities, including the development of regional centers of excellence and services not offered by either system; to attract physicians, nurses, and other health professionals; to expand education and medical training programs; and to promote economic development in the region. Expansion of Sanford Health's market area into North Dakota is also expected to reduce the outmigration of patients to other markets, and the combined financial position should improve access

to capital needed to fund strategic initiatives. This merger will also expand research opportunities and help medical schools in the Dakotas collaborate on training and residency programs to retain more graduates in the region (Sanford Health–MeritCare 2009b).

The partnership between Advocate Health Care and BroMenn, completed in January 2010, is another arrangement expected to yield significant community benefits. In late 2008, Advocate Health Care, the largest healthcare provider in Illinois, had more than 200 sites in metropolitan Chicago, including eight acute care hospitals, two children's hospitals, and a large medical group (Advocate Health Care 2010). Before the end of 2008, Advocate acquired a ninth hospital situated in a northern suburb of Chicago. Three months earlier, Advocate had approached BroMenn Healthcare System, located 130 miles southwest of Chicago in the central Illinois city of Bloomington, about a potential partnership (BroMenn Healthcare 2008).

The opportunity was attractive to BroMenn, a two-hospital system with 11 medical practices, because the organizations share a mission of providing community healthcare with faith-based roots, excellent reputations for clinical care, and a commitment to working in partnership with physicians. For Advocate, this first partnership outside of Chicago is a significant step toward its vision of a statewide health system (Advocate Health Care 2009).

The University of Pittsburgh Medical Center (UPMC), which has completed more than a dozen mergers/acquisitions over three decades, has a vision of community change on a grand scale. UPMC has transformed itself from a loose federation of six hospitals into a multibillion-dollar global health enterprise with 20 hospitals, 400 outpatient sites, a 1.4 million member health plan, and a clinical presence in multiple international markets. Its early vision was to create a leading-edge healthcare system in western Pennsylvania and transform the economy in Pittsburgh and throughout the region. Today, UPMC's vision is to create a new economic future for western Pennsylvania by exporting excellence nationally and internationally. To achieve this vision, UPMC plans to develop new businesses to commercialize its expertise, to continue to make significant investments in new fields of medical research, and to implement information technol-

ogy capable of integrating care settings (UPMC 2009a, 2009b, 2009c).

CONCLUSION

The rationale for combining two organizations is a statement that guides the discussions and important decisions following the proposal of a merger or acquisition. While the benefits of a merger or acquisition, such as the potential for growth, financial stability, and higher-quality, more accessible patient care, may seem tangible and obvious to the executives and boards participating in the discussions, the rationale, as expressed in the vision statement, will communicate this message internally and externally. Many constituents, particularly those outside of the organizations, will come to understand the need for the merger or acquisition only through expression of the organizations' shared vision. The vision statement will also provide a reference point for future decision making, as the complicated initial stages of the merger process unfold.

CHAPTER 1 KEY TAKEAWAYS

- It is imperative to start the merger process with a clear sense of what (at a high level) is to be accomplished because it will be tested frequently.

- The underlying rationale for the merger must describe higher purposes and significant benefits that the merging organizations can realize collectively but not on their own.

- The rationale should describe a preferred future state that is ten or more years away and represent a stretch target that motivates, energizes, and inspires the combining organizations to attain it.

- The primary elements of the rationale usually include opportunities for growth, better performance, and improved finances as well as tangible community benefits, such as more local health-care options and new economic development.

- For many constituents, particularly those outside of the two organizations and the rank and file within them, the vision is likely to be the way they come to understand the need for the transaction, so it should be a central feature in both internal and external communications about the merger or acquisition.

CHAPTER 2

Cultural Compatibility

PETER V. MCGINN

Struggling hospitals and health systems often look to mergers as the silver bullet to success, but this strategy sometimes fails to deliver the promised magic. A major mistake in premerger assessments is attention to only a subset of relevant factors. As one chief operating officer of a major health system who has negotiated a number of mergers and acquisitions explained, "Culture usually gets second billing behind financial measures."

Mergers are like marriages; even the premerger and "courtship" processes are similar. Participants often do not ask important questions or have meaningful discussions at this stage. In some regards, premerger discussions resemble premarital conversations observed by marriage counselors. The betrothed, deeply in love, have problems that are obvious to many third-party observers, but explicit recognition of those problems might threaten the likelihood of proceeding with the wedding. The couple makes a choice that some merging businesses have made—they cease the assessment and go ahead with their plans. This chapter describes a better approach to premerger discussion, offering principles, tools, and categories useful in evaluating the compatibility of the merger candidates' values and culture.

In affiliation discussions, financial and service line factors typically receive the attention they deserve because financial distress or financial goals are often the driving factors in mergers and acquisitions. Without perceived financial or market benefits, there would be no impulse for such proposals. Accordingly, examination of balance sheets, cost and debt structures, earnings and margin, forecasts, geographic markets, and compensation and benefits structure is essential. This information forms the business justification for many mergers and acquisitions.

These factors are obvious because they are necessary. If a proposed merger does not make sense from a financial or market point of view, it should not be pursued. Few boards or management teams overlook these factors, although occasionally, the promise of a financial rescue or the lure of synergy is so strong that otherwise sensible people forget to exercise due diligence.

As important as these factors are, they are insufficient to adequately assess a potential merger partner. Organizations have histories. Like people, they have personalities or, as they are called in business, cultures. Merger partners are not likely to be identical, but they do need to be compatible. Thus, a cultural assessment is also necessary.

COMPONENTS OF A PREMERGER CULTURAL ASSESSMENT

Like personalities, organizational cultures are multidimensional. Which cultural factors will have the greatest impact on the outcome of a merger? There is no single right answer, but there are nine areas that should be part of any premerger assessment:

1. Abilities and other intangible assets
2. Core values
3. Communication styles
4. Decision-making styles
5. Expectations
6. Financial indicators

7. Human resources philosophy and systems
8. Incentives
9. Accountability

Abilities and Other Intangible Assets

What special talents or other intangible assets exist in each organization? Will corporate politics waste or overlook the talents of the people originally working for the non-dominant partner? Will the partners be able to merge their strengths? Will they be able to overcome their weaknesses?

Core Values

What drives the organizations? What are their implicit and explicit criteria for success? Values do not have to match for merged organizations to achieve success, but values must lead to compatible actions or the merged organizations will flounder and suffer false starts. Incompatibility of values often leads to distrust and lack of mutual respect.

Communication Styles

Communication styles are often taken for granted. People typically view their organization's style as the way things should be done. How does management communicate? How open or closed are communica-

tion channels? How much is communicated by rumor? Is information hoarded or shared? Are the formal channels accurate? Are they trusted? Does information flow up, down, or sideways? How much information is filtered? What information is protected?

Decision-Making Styles

When two organizations' decision-making styles do not match, the gears of the combined system cease to grind smoothly. How are important decisions made, and who participates in these decisions? What type of evidence is required to support a decision? How many sign-offs or approvals are required to make a decision official? What are the organizations' risk thresholds? Do the organizations have a predisposition toward being highly skeptical and cautious versus ambitious and open-minded?

Expectations

What expectations do the organizations have regarding the strategy, benefits, and negative consequences of the merger? Both organizations' stated and unstated expectations need to be tested. They are likely to be different, but that is okay. Partners can enter the relationship for different reasons. For example, one may be looking for a financial lifeline, while the other is looking for a shortcut into a new market. Trouble arises when neither side understands the rewards the other is seeking.

Financial Indicators

How does each organization define financial success? For example, does it stress profitability, cash, revenue growth, or earnings before interest, taxes, depreciation, and amortization? Each party should be aware of the other's preferred measure and consider which measures will be most appropriate for the combined venture.

Human Resources Philosophy and Systems

Do the organizations invest in employee and management development? Merging organizations must determine whether their potential partner views people as assets or expenses. An organization that runs according to tight productivity formulas will clash with an organization that is more casual about staffing levels. An organization that spends a lot of resources on employee recognition will not mesh with one that cuts such spending. An organization that emphasizes shared

values will recoil at an organization that stresses individual achievement and individual rewards.

Incentives

How do the organizations reward their employees? The incentives an organization uses reveal much about that organization's understanding of its employees and their motivations. An organization oriented around monetary incentives may be incompatible with one oriented around small or intangible rewards. Employees caught in the middle of a merger involving organizations offering dissimilar incentives are likely to feel confused, manipulated, and disillusioned.

Accountability

Are people held accountable for performance? How regularly is performance measured and tracked? Does accountability differ according to organizational level? Some organizations assess performance globally and qualitatively, while others are more specific and quantitative in their approach. Some stress team performance, while others track individual accomplishments. An organization with an individual performance/reward culture will not mesh easily with an organization that has a "we are family; all do well or all do poorly" perspective.

COMPATIBILITY OF VALUES

Potential partners have to look beyond appearances to assess the compatibility of their values. Typical value statements express generic good behaviors and positive intentions. Using these statements as a stimulus for better organizational performance may be appropriate, but using them as a guide for evaluating actual organizational values is risky.

Lencioni (2002) suggested a four-part categorization of values:

1. **Core values**—the deeply ingrained principles that guide behavior in an organization, such as "the HP Way"
2. **Aspirational values**—characteristics an organization values, but currently lacks, such as boldness or excellence
3. **"Permission-to-play" values**—values that are not distinctive but are minimal standards expected of any organization, such as integrity
4. **Accidental values**—values an organization developed through its

history but that are not essential to its success, such as deference to an inner circle of leaders

A fifth category should also be considered:

5. **Counterfeit values**—values claimed by an organization, but not actually practiced, such as Enron's supposed values of respect, integrity, communication, and excellence

There is often a difference between values in practice and values in principle. When asked to identify their values, people/organizations color their answers with a social desirability factor. In other words, people express values that reflect well on them and support their self-image and self-esteem. A better way to identify their values is to observe behavior. A typical assessment, whether done internally or with the assistance of a third party, would begin with an examination of such indicators as

- written organizational values;
- past decisions;
- implicit or explicit decision rules;
- reactions to opportunities, problems, and crises;
- conflicts;

- priorities reflected in budgets and plans;
- policies and exceptions to policies; and
- stories, legends, heroes, stars, and villains.

Some of these indicators are obvious, while others are subtle and more difficult to discern. A better understanding of an organization's values can be gained through an assessment of all these indicators than through consideration of only one indicator, such as stated values.

A four-point model for categorizing the results of a values assessment between organizations is shown in Exhibit 2.1. This helpful tool recognizes that not all results will fit in a single category. At least three of the four are likely to apply.

Values need not be identical for an affiliation to succeed. The merger of two organizations with different but compatible values may strengthen both organizations. For example, if Organization X is passionate about its mission but somewhat tentative in decision making, it may benefit from a partnership with a more confident organization. If the more confident organization has a history of inconsistent action because it is less attached to a mis-sion or vision, it may benefit from Organization X's increased clarity of purpose and become less reactive. Conflicting values, however, will undermine the benefits of a merger if they are not recognized and reconciled.

ENGAGING THE BOARD AND TOP MANAGEMENT IN DISCUSSIONS ABOUT VALUES

An effective way to begin a cultural assessment is to initiate discussions with cross-organizational planning teams comprising board members and top management. Adjective checklists and comparable devices facilitate dialogue and are productive tools to use during these discussions. They are especially useful in discussions about sensitive topics. Discussion within organizations is often as critical as the discussion between organizations, so both should be encouraged and fostered.

Organizations usually are not as different as they think they are and often detect more similarities than they expected. Where conflicts are identified, a safe and open environment should be created for exploring definitions, considering compromises, and testing limits.

EXHIBIT 2.1: Four-Point Scale for Categorizing Results of a Values Assessment

Consistent or comparable	The same, or essentially the same
Compatible	Different, but fit together without conflict
Complementary	Different, but produce a positive effect when combined
Conflicting	Inconsistent; problematic if not reconciled

CULTURAL INCOMPATIBILITY AND COMPATIBILITY IN THE REAL WORLD: WHAT IT LOOKS LIKE

In the early 1990s, Pennsylvania State University Hershey Medical Center and Geisinger Health System in Danville, Pennsylvania, explored a possible affiliation on two separate occasions but neither process identified significant opportunities. A small working group began a third round of discussions in the spring of 1996, and the boards of both organizations unanimously approved a merger in January 1997. Less than three years later, both boards voted unanimously to unwind the merger, citing cultural incompatibility as the main driver of the dissolution (Mallon 2003).

At the time of the merger, the components needed to ensure a successful combination appeared to be in place. The healthcare environment was characterized by the spread of managed care, the creation of integrated delivery systems, and the threat of reduced Medicare reimbursement. Both Penn State and Geisinger were nonprofit, physician-led groups with missions centered on patient care, education, and research, and both had roots in philanthropy. Strengthened clinical enterprises, improved market position, and savings were the expected outcomes of the merger. The organizations' leaders noted these commonalities early on, but as the merger proceeded, they discovered that the organizations' priorities were out of sync. Penn State was committed to preserving and maintaining its academic mission and the financial viability of its College of Medicine, while Geisinger's primary aim was to expand its health plan to find new markets for its clinical services (Mallon 2003).

Incompatibilities were also evident in the emphasis each placed on the three mission areas of patient care, education, and research. As a classical group practice, Geisinger's focus was largely on patient care, while Penn State, an academic health center, was balancing patient care relatively equally with its commitments to education and research. Furthermore, both organizations valued participatory management, but their underlying assumptions about this approach were different (Mallon 2003).

Unlike Penn State and Geisinger, BJC HealthCare, based in St. Louis, surmounted major cultural challenges at its outset and during its development and now thrives as a local, regional, and national leader in healthcare delivery, taking in approximately $3.5 billion in annual revenue. BJC, one of the largest not-for-profit healthcare organizations in the United States, is the product of multiple linkages. A Jewish-sponsored hospital merged with a nonsectarian hospital (that had religious roots), and then the combined organization, Barnes-Jewish, Inc., merged with Christian Hospital, a faith-based organization

affiliated with the Christian Women's Benevolent Association. BJC proceeded to blend with the academic-based organizations affiliated with the Washington University School of Medicine—all located on one campus, along with many community-based organizations. As a result, BJC has become a uniquely American melting pot (Lipstein 2009).

Unlike other organizations that had attempted similar mergers, BJC HealthCare succeeded. How did they do it? Steven H. Lipstein, who became BJC's second CEO and president in 1999, says the key has been maintaining a balance between the community and academic cultures and other potentially disparate cultural elements. BJC's leadership made balance a guiding principle and did not let one culture dominate the others (Lipstein 2009).

The following data, which pertain to the last ten years, demonstrate this balance (Lipstein 2009):

- The academic-related institutions generated 50.1 percent of total net revenues, and the community-based organizations and other institutions generated the remaining 49.9 percent.
- Forty-nine percent of total earnings before interest, depreciation,

and amortization is attributable to the academic-related institutions, and the remaining 51 percent is attributable to the community-based organizations and other institutions.

- The academic-related institutions accounted for 52.6 percent of capital expenditures, and 47.4 percent went to the community-based organizations and other institutions.

BJC continues to be a learning organization with an unusually strong commitment to the growth and development of its employees. About 2,000 of BJC's 26,000 employees are enrolled in next-step education at any one time. Continuous improvement and progress toward one culture are important by-products of this commitment (Lipstein 2009).

CONCLUSION

The history of mergers and acquisitions shows that lack of cultural compatibility between combining organizations is one of the most frequent obstacles to mergers and their subsequent success. A premerger cultural compatibility assessment is as important as premerger financial, market, and operational assessments. The nine assessment categories identified in this chapter are essential considerations in such an evaluation. Comparison of values is not the only important part of this assessment, but it is a good starting point and a means of engaging the board and top management in formative discussions.

Mergers are a sound strategic answer for many organizations facing difficult competitive situations. They can strengthen finances, market position, and operational capabilities. When potential partners do not consider cultural compatibility from the beginning of the process, however, they often end up suboptimizing the opportunities and potential they had envisioned.

CHAPTER 2 KEY TAKEAWAYS

- Organizations evaluating a merger or acquisition tend to focus on whether the combination makes sense from a financial or market point of view and overlook the importance of cultural fit. Partners do not need to be identical, but they should be compatible.
- To gain an understanding of the multidimensional aspects

of culture, organizations should conduct a premerger or acquisition assessment that looks at nine areas: abilities and other intangible assets, core values, communication styles, decision-making styles, expectations, financial indicators, human resources philosophy and systems, incentives, and accountability.

- Potential merger or affiliation partners must look beyond the typical value statements that express generic good behaviors and positive intentions and examine five categories of values: core values, aspirational values, "permission-to-play" values, accidental values, and counterfeit values.

- Values need not be identical for an affiliation to succeed. Different but compatible values may strengthen both organizations. Conflicting values, however, will undermine the benefits of a merger if they are not recognized and reconciled.

- An effective approach to begin a cultural assessment is to initiate discussions with cross-organizational planning teams comprising board members and top management. Discussion within organizations may be as critical as the discussion between organizations, so both should be encouraged and fostered. Where conflicts are identified, a safe and open environment should be created for exploring definitions, considering compromises, and testing limits.

CHAPTER 3

Governance

KEITH T. PRYOR

Nothing derails a merger more quickly than a sloppy conversation about governance. Governance may not seem like a topic that needs to be addressed sensitively, but it does. It encompasses almost all that is precarious in the high-wire and high-level discussions that take place among the principals involved in a merger: ego, control, history, style, personality, structure, timing, and money.

Too many executives and board leaders view governance as primarily about structure. In a merger, it is usually better for those involved to appreciate that governance discussions are mostly about trade-offs, and those trade-offs usually involve people and their (often) all too personal goals. Structural detail comes up further down the road.

Regardless of whether the organization is an acquiring entity, an acquired entity, or something in between, rarely does it gain all that it desires in a merger agreement. Mergers involve negotiation, and every negotiation involves trade-offs. One thing is certain: The other side will see things differently, even if the organizations are compatible and have compelling reasons to consolidate.

Ultimately, the board will decide whether the affiliation will take place. In some situations, the board drives the affiliation process. Consequently, board leadership will play a seminal role in affiliation discussions, and most, if not all, of what follows in this chapter applies to board leadership as well as CEOs. That said, CEOs tend to play the lead role in advancing affiliation discussions, so the chapter focuses on their efforts.

Given the sensitivity of the subjects involved in negotiations and trade-offs, executives participating in merger governance discussions should be well prepared, particularly in these five areas:

1. The A-game
2. The right people
3. History
4. Goals
5. Structure

THE A-GAME

The demands placed on the CEOs and board leadership involved in merger discussions are enormous, although the CEOs bear the brunt of it. Stress is everywhere—in the prolonged negotiations requiring intense concentration, in the wake of criticism from those who have limited appreciation for the complexity of the task, and in mixed-motive deliberations—and all the while the trains need to be kept running on time. It is such a high-adrenaline period that many CEOs experience a significant decline in energy when merger negotiations are complete.

To deal with this pressure, CEOs involved in merger governance discussions need to be at the top of their game. By following these guidelines, they can optimize their readiness for the task ahead:

■ This work will take extra time—meaning nights and weekends that are not already taken up. Take care of yourself physically and mentally. Get adequate sleep and exercise, eat well, and plan time off—mergers always take longer than anticipated.

- A discussion with your family may be in order. You will want them to understand and support the professional demands you will experience and appreciate that there will be an end date. Depending on the nature of the merger, you may want to prepare them for controversy and resulting media attention, not all of which will be flattering.

- Think through and assess your strengths and weaknesses. Expect your strengths to be tested. Expect your soft spots to be exposed and perhaps exploited, and plan accordingly.

- If you believe that your political skills have never been sharp, keep close counsel with someone whose skills are. If you are not as quick with a balance sheet as you would like to be, keep your chief financial officer nearby.

- Know that life will not be the same when the merger agreement is complete. You may be exhilarated, or you may be bored. You may feel a great deal has been accomplished; you may feel that your new job is underwhelming. You will likely not be able to predict the outcome, but be prepared for your world to be dramatically different when the process is complete.

THE RIGHT PEOPLE

A board steering committee will be needed to deal with the governance aspects of the merger. CEOs are inclined to select the three to five trustees who will serve on this committee from among their officers or executive committee. That may be the way to go, but what is most important is that they be the right *people*, not necessarily the people in the right *positions*. Keep these competencies and experiences in mind:

- **Experience counts**. Trustees who have been through a merger, possibly in their own industry, can be invaluable. They often have an appreciation for pace, are not overly affected by minor mishaps along the way, and can bring a certain gravitas to the work.

- **Interpersonal skills are paramount**. The merger process is mainly about interpersonal skills, so the steering committee should have them and, hopefully, contained egos. During the opening "get to know you" period of a merger planning session, I once listened to a trustee explain the extensive and detailed financial support his hospital would require if it were acquired by a larger, more successful system. It was painful to watch enthusiasm for the merger melt from the faces of the larger system's representatives as the trustee clumsily laid out his demands.

■ **Big-picture people excel at merger work**. Effective merger steering committee members can see their way through small glitches, make requests that cost more than anticipated but are warranted, and make compromises that their organization would prefer not to make—all with an eye on the prize, understanding that they may not see results for several years.

■ **Credibility is a big help during merger transactions**. Merger discussions do not always proceed smoothly. In the worst case, they can fall apart, publicly and quickly. Steering committee members should command respect within and outside the organization.

■ **Do not forget the physicians**. Physicians are overlooked more often than one might think, and it never goes over well. As discussed in more detail in Chapter 5, a respected physician must be part of merger discussions from the beginning. He or she needs to be able to communicate effectively to the medical staff or members of the group practice about the goals and status of the merger discussions when appropriate. A medical staff steering committee working in tandem with the board-level committee may also be needed during hospital mergers.

HISTORY

The merger team or board steering committee needs to take time to understand the potential partner's relevant history, including past relationships between the organizations, important events, and key individuals. Mergers are marriages of sorts, and the vows will be easier spoken if there is a sense that each party knows the other as well as possible. An awareness of relevant history is also a strong antidote against major faux pas during the sensitive discussions that occur during merger transactions.

A case involving three independent hospitals in western Massachusetts highlights the importance of gaining a sense of the history between organizations. Two of the three hospitals had joined together and formed a strong, sophisticated system in the Berkshires. Although the third hospital was aware that its future would likely be limited as an independent facility, it turned down the system's repeated invitations to join, having long felt slighted by the system's hospitals. When a new CEO from the community arrived at the large system, the competitive landscape changed dramatically. The new CEO understood the history between the organizations and appreciated the position and legacy of the third hospital. A short time after his arrival, the hospital joined the system.

GOALS

Sometimes the goals that brought the organizations to the negotiating table drop out of sight after two meetings about governance and are replaced by misunderstood history, bruised egos, angry board members, and hardened negotiating positions. To avoid this situation, organizations considering a merger should know the goals up front and find ways to refresh everyone's mind about them throughout the process. Every merger is different, but the list of goals may encompass some or all of the following:

- Commitment to the community and maintaining appropriate levels of service
- Expanded range of service offerings and market depth
- Better financial performance and balance sheet strength
- Ability to do more (e.g., recruit specialists) than can be done now
- Quality improvement
- Defense against other competitors

Goals do not include determining such details as how many members will serve on the new board or who the new CEO will be. As critical as the resolution of these and similar issues are to the ultimate success of the merger (see below), these decisions are just steps along the way. A successful merger evolves from clarity about the larger goals of the venture, which tend to be results oriented and community centered.

STRUCTURE

Compared to the overall complexity of merger transactions, governance structure issues are not that complicated. Well-researched resources describing alternative approaches to governance models are available. Many CEOs may feel they already have a sense of the possibilities. Important factors in structure discussions often boil down to three broad subject areas: leadership, timetable for integration of governance systems, and control and design.

Leadership

The question of who is to be appointed CEO is best addressed early on. Early appointment may seem premature and impractical, but if this issue remains open, it will color all subsequent discussions. It can be resolved early on via a meeting of the current CEOs or by the board chairs, but it needs to be addressed. There are only three options:

1. One of the CEOs becomes the CEO of the merged entity, and the other either resigns or takes another position in the merged organization, which may pose its own risks and challenges.
2. Both CEOs resign, and the organizations recruit a new one.
3. A search takes place and one or the other CEO vies for the posi-

tion, which is nearly as bad as not addressing the issue at all.

The appointment of a new board chair is also a potent topic, sometimes as critical as the CEO question, but usually less volatile. Unless the merger is a board-driven process, the CEO question needs to be resolved before the question of board leadership in the new organization can be raised.

Timetable

Governance literature generally agrees that nonrepresentational governance is an important component of effective multi-organizational governance. Boards that include "three trustees from organization A and four from organization B . . ." have a difficult time operating as an integrated entity. The best boards of merged entities operate in such a way that an objective observer would not discern bias from any trustee toward either organization.

Why not design an unbiased, integrated board for the new entity? Sometimes it cannot be done. In some cases, a system of limited representation (i.e., fewer board members from the organization that is merging into the other), at least for a few years, eases conflict and enables trustees to move forward with a merger that is ultimately a good thing for the community.

A frank discussion, early on, of the value of nonrepresentational governance and setting a timetable for getting there are valuable parts of merger governance discussions. This process can take a few years. Develop a plan, and designate a board of no more than 20 members; if too many voices are involved, the new organization may never get to where it is planning to go.

Control and Design

CEOs are likely to give up more control in governance discussions than expected. Potential merger partners may require more seats than the CEO thinks they deserve. Concessions may need to be made to keep the merger moving forward. What CEOs and their steering committees should not do, however, is create an ungainly governance model that cannot accomplish the goals that have been set. For example, if quality improvement is essential and it is best accomplished via a system-level quality committee that drives quality down and throughout the organization, an extra seat or two on that quality committee may need to be conceded to the other party; however, the structure of the committee should remain unchanged so that quality continues to be led at the organizational level.

Similarly, concessions on reserved powers, while occasionally necessary, should be made with great caution, as these powers, more than structure itself, concern strategy and leadership philosophy. While sometimes useful, advisory boards incorporated as a way of accommodating the less powerful party's wishes to remain involved in governance can become a political nuisance, adding little value while using extensive board and leadership time and energy to quell minor fires, respond to small-scale issues, and satisfy the discontented. Advisory committees are often a better choice.

SIMPLICITY The prevailing thinking on governance design is that simpler is better. Simpler means as few boards as possible and optimizing and pruning standing committees to the least number necessary to do the work of the board. In complex integrated systems, the most effective boards are those whose power is largely centralized and for which trustees are chosen not on the basis of the organizations they represent but their ability to bring critical capabilities, breadth, and regional and strategic thinking to the system. In an affiliation, that generally means striving for the smallest governance structure possible.

TriHealth, a sophisticated system in Cincinnati, Ohio, is especially skilled and diligent in its commitment to as simple a governance structure as possible, even though the original organization was rather complex—the joining of a Catholic provider (which was already part of a national Catholic system) and a strong secular community hospital. As the organization has expanded, the governance structure has remained largely intact; the parent governing body sets strategy and goals and drives performance throughout the system.

Again, be clear on the goals of the merger and how those goals would be best accomplished. Create a structure that supports achievement of those goals. Compromise on membership and involvement, but do not compromise on structure and power if doing so will impede the achievement of what the merging organizations have set out to do.

CONCLUSION

Mergers involve intricate, high-level discussions that lead to major transformational decisions. While governance decisions may not rank highly among the many complex issues that need to be addressed, they must be handled with sensitivity and an appreciation that negotiations and trade-offs are likely to dominate discussions more so than issues related to structure. CEOs and board leadership involved in merger transactions will need to focus on having their A-game, assembling the right people, being sensitive to history, setting clear goals, and creating a sensible structure. All the rest is discussion, negotiation, and trade-offs.

CHAPTER 3 KEY TAKEAWAYS

- Governance must be addressed sensitively because it involves the potentially volatile issues of ego, control, history, style, personality, structure, timing, and money.
- CEOs and board leadership need to be at the top of their game to manage the prolonged stress of merger negotiations, including being self-aware about strengths

and weaknesses, particularly political skills.

- The board steering committee addressing governance issues related
to the mergers should comprise
the right *people*, not the people in
the right *positions*.

- Awareness of the relevant histories each organization brings to
the merger discussions will help
minimize gaffes during sensitive
discussions.

- The original goals of the affiliation should be referred to
often as the merger discussions
proceed and complexities cloud
the original intentions of the
merger.

- Discussions about governance
structure should address leadership (both CEO and board chair
positions), a timetable for integration of governance systems,
and control.

Organization and Operating Structure

SAMUEL H. STEINBERG,

ALAN M. ZUCKERMAN, AND

MICHAEL J. WALTERS

Healthcare mergers present challenging decisions that will have lasting effects on the new organization. Many of these decisions relate to the organizational and operating structure. The most pressing concern in early merger discussions often is appointment of those who will be in charge and in control, but equally important is the design of the new organization. The way the new organization will be structured and operated will determine its eventual success or failure and touch the lives of everyone it employs.

Newly merged organizations often fail to achieve the premerger goals they set. The typical merged entity moves quickly to achieve economies of scale from coordinated purchasing of goods and services and may pursue other savings in administrative activities, such as combining legal services or consolidating contract service companies. Higher-achieving organizations eliminate duplicative management staff, hopefully in a respectful manner. Few new post-merger entities take on the challenges of reorganizing patient care services and processes right away, even though this area may yield the greatest potential benefits.

This chapter provides guidance on how to design, organize, and operate the new entity so that the organization meets the goals of the merger and achieves its highest potential. Merger planning at this stage usually yields three critical outputs:

- Overall corporate structure
- High-level organizational and operational framework
- Supporting leadership structure

The process of determining the organizational and operating structure is more art than science and influenced as much by negotiation among the leadership of the combining entities as by rational needs. It is also iterative (sometimes even circular), and the solution often emerges after both leadership groups reach exhaustion.

OVERALL CORPORATE STRUCTURE

The question to be answered here is: What form is necessary and desired to achieve the functional ends of the proposed relationship? While form should follow function, many healthcare deals address form before function and then attempt to retrofit, often with great difficulty, the functions and intended benefits/ends to an inconsistent form/structure.

Exhibit 4.1 illustrates the typical relationship between form and function/benefit under various types of affiliations, as well as the influence of culture on both. The chart shows that

- there are five broad categories (and many subcategories) of corporate forms of affiliation, ranging from loose strategic alliances to tight asset mergers; and
- organizations that are tightly structured, are highly interdependent, and have high cultural compatibility generally reap the greatest performance and financial benefits.

Per the focus of this book, this chapter concentrates on the joint

EXHIBIT 4.1: Healthcare Organizational Design in Affiliated Entities: Form Versus Function

POTENTIAL FINANCIAL
IMPACT

Limited · Extensive

Tight Most Important

Asset
Merger

INTERDEPENDENCE

Shared Service
Organization

Joint Operating
Agreement (JOA)

CULTURAL COMPATIBILITY

Strategic
Alliance

Service-Specific
Joint Venture

Loose Least Important

Limited POTENTIAL IMPACT ON TOTAL Extensive
ORGANIZATIONAL PERFORMANCE

SOURCE: Copyright Health Strategies & Solutions, Inc. (2010). Used with permission.

operating agreement and asset merger structures.

While the choice between the joint operating agreement and asset merger structures may appear straightforward, it often is not. The desire to optimize benefits is usually clear, but interdependence and cultural factors may constrain benefits realization. The desire on the part of one or both organizations for some degree of autonomy is often a concern and may be a primary topic in governance discussions. Joint operating agreements have been used most frequently in mergers of Catholic and non-Catholic organizations as a means of preserving some degree of separation to avoid church-related problems. Differences in organizations' cultures and operating styles are the other barrier to full integration. To surmount this barrier, the organizations may decide to implement a phased plan for full integration or settle for a structure short of total assimilation as a way to balance competing concerns. Key trade-offs and implications of these organizational structure alternatives are further illustrated in exhibits 4.2, 4.3, and 4.4.

In October 2008, two systems primarily serving northern Kentucky— St. Elizabeth Medical Center, Inc., a Catholic health system, and St. Luke Hospitals, Inc., a nonreligious, community hospital system—merged into a single entity, with St. Elizabeth Healthcare as the surviving nonprofit corporation. Competitive factors and the experiences of both organizations in affiliations with larger Cincinnati health systems were key considerations that led to the choice of a single nonprofit corporation as the structure for the new organization. Both organizations had been in loose alliances in which neither party received sufficient value to offset the control they relinquished. For example, St. Elizabeth joined Catholic Healthcare Partners in 1998 as an affiliate and found after four years that

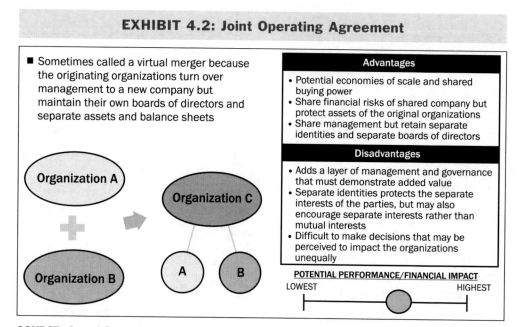

EXHIBIT 4.2: Joint Operating Agreement

- Sometimes called a virtual merger because the originating organizations turn over management to a new company but maintain their own boards of directors and separate assets and balance sheets

Advantages
- Potential economies of scale and shared buying power
- Share financial risks of shared company but protect assets of the original organizations
- Share management but retain separate identities and separate boards of directors

Disadvantages
- Adds a layer of management and governance that must demonstrate added value
- Separate identities protects the separate interests of the parties, but may also encourage separate interests rather than mutual interests
- Difficult to make decisions that may be perceived to impact the organizations unequally

Organization A + Organization B → Organization C (A, B)

POTENTIAL PERFORMANCE/FINANCIAL IMPACT
LOWEST   HIGHEST

EXHIBIT 4.3: Parent/Holding Company (One Type of Full Asset Merger)

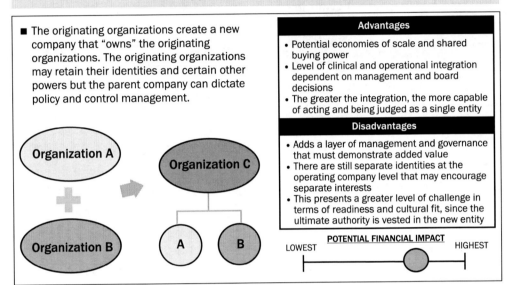

- The originating organizations create a new company that "owns" the originating organizations. The originating organizations may retain their identities and certain other powers but the parent company can dictate policy and control management.

Advantages

- Potential economies of scale and shared buying power
- Level of clinical and operational integration dependent on management and board decisions
- The greater the integration, the more capable of acting and being judged as a single entity

Disadvantages

- Adds a layer of management and governance that must demonstrate added value
- There are still separate identities at the operating company level that may encourage separate interests
- This presents a greater level of challenge in terms of readiness and cultural fit, since the ultimate authority is vested in the new entity

POTENTIAL FINANCIAL IMPACT
LOWEST   HIGHEST

SOURCE: Copyright Health Strategies & Solutions, Inc. (2010). Used with permission.

EXHIBIT 4.4: Full Asset Merger

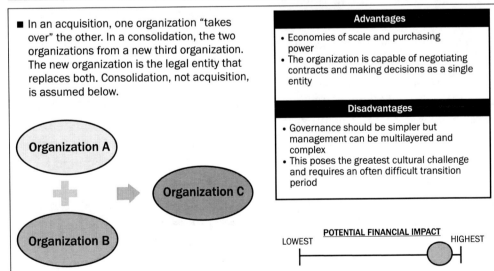

- In an acquisition, one organization "takes over" the other. In a consolidation, the two organizations from a new third organization. The new organization is the legal entity that replaces both. Consolidation, not acquisition, is assumed below.

Advantages

- Economies of scale and purchasing power
- The organization is capable of negotiating contracts and making decisions as a single entity

Disadvantages

- Governance should be simpler but management can be multilayered and complex
- This poses the greatest cultural challenge and requires an often difficult transition period

POTENTIAL FINANCIAL IMPACT
LOWEST   HIGHEST

SOURCE: Copyright Health Strategies & Solutions, Inc. (2010). Used with permission.

there were insufficient synergies with Mercy Health Partners of Southwest Ohio, another member of Catholic Healthcare Partners, to tolerate the increasing demands for centralization and system control. St. Luke's board, which had chosen to join the Health Alliance of Greater Cincinnati in 1995, felt increasingly that the Alliance was making capital allocation decisions that overwhelmingly favored the hospitals in southwest Ohio over the hospitals in northern Kentucky, where the St. Luke facilities were located.

As St. Luke was attempting to merge with St. Elizabeth, it was embroiled in a messy separation from the Health Alliance, an entity structured as a joint operating agreement since its formation in 1993. The departure of St. Luke from the Health Alliance in 2008 after years of bitter financial and legal battles was a contributing factor in the dissolution of the Health Alliance, which at one time was the largest healthcare provider in the greater Cincinnati area. These events in the greater Cincinnati market clearly demonstrate that loose affiliations eventually blow apart, and when they do, the divorces are ugly and painful.

The St. Elizabeth–St. Luke merger involved unequal partners. Regardless of the statistic, measure, or ratio considered, St. Elizabeth was the stronger, financially healthier organization. St. Elizabeth's negotiating team asserted early in the merger discussions that it was critical to create a single entity that could not be pulled apart. Rather than create an entirely new third organization, St. Luke disappeared as a corporate entity and only St. Elizabeth remained. However, the final merger agreement did not propose new names for the St. Luke facilities and stated that a supermajority vote of the new board would be required to make any such changes.

HIGH-LEVEL ORGANIZATIONAL AND OPERATIONAL FRAMEWORK

Once consensus has been reached on the form of the combined organization, the next level of structure design—the design and functions of executive management and its relationship to, as well as the high-level relationships among, business units, service lines, and other key corporate entities—must be addressed. Goals of the merger partners will guide the development of this design. Common goals that influence the design of merged organizations include

- the ability to support strategy,
- effective and efficient use of resources,
- streamlined decision making,
- synergy among operating units and reduction of silos, and
- specific desired results in such areas as clinical quality; financial targets; and employee, physician, and patient satisfaction.

High-level organizational and operational design is also influenced by local, regional, and state market focus and factors, particularly competition, the payer environment, the medical practice environment, and legal, regulatory, and political constraints. In conceptualizing any new organizational and operational design, four critical variables and potential trade-offs must be considered:

1. **Centralized versus decentralized**. Will significant authority be vested in the corporate office, or will the operating units have greater autonomy and responsibility for profit and loss? Will staff functions be located at corporate or in the operating units? Will systems and processes be standardized across operating units? To what degree?

2. **Flat/broad versus narrow/deep**. Will generalists manage business broadly and emphasize teamwork and cross-functional cooperation, or will the organization emphasize specialization with narrow functional responsibilities and service lines that run relatively independently of each other? Will depth and breadth vary across the system?

3. **Product/service compatibility**. What products and services can be coupled to build efficiencies and other synergies in the structure? This choice will be heavily influenced by the market as well as the type and characteristics of products and services offered.

4. **Functions and value of each management layer**. Identifying expected responsibilities and authority, as well as the value added by each management layer, provides a level of design rigor missing in most organizations.

The result of these analyses and associated deliberations is a schematic and outline of relationships among senior and middle management levels as well as important subcomponents of the new organization, and associated guiding operations concepts and principles.

For an example of how these discussions play out in real-world situations, consider once more the St. Elizabeth–St. Luke merger case. Both parties believed St. Elizabeth to be the dominant and more successful health system. In the merger discussions, they agreed that St. Elizabeth's CEO would be the CEO of the new entity. The CEO and his senior management team determined that the initial structure of the organization should be centralized for two key reasons. First, all the facilities in the merged organization would serve essentially the same market. Leadership viewed the determination of services to be provided in each area as system decisions, not the domain of individual facilities, particularly because opportunities for consolidation and cost efficiencies were substantial across the system. Second, before the merger, St. Luke provided few corporate-type services for itself, such as revenue cycle management, information systems, and human resources. Instead, a centralized Health Alliance corporate office provided these services. Consequently, prior to the merger, St. Luke's management team was minimal and em-

phasized the management of clinical departments.

To provide consistent, on-site senior leadership, a COO from St. Elizabeth's senior ranks was immediately assigned to each St. Luke hospital. A senior vice president was assigned to each functional area of the organization and asked to develop a structure for his or her division. One fairly consistent outcome of this approach was that system-wide positions for management of functions across all sites were generally, but not exclusively, filled from within. The rationale for this structural design was the need to maximize cooperation, execute cost efficiencies quickly, and expedite the development of a unified culture across the organization.

SUPPORTING LEADERSHIP STRUCTURE

The nuts and bolts of organizational structure are the arrangement of boxes with names or positions in an organizational chart to reflect pragmatic issues of day-to-day functionality. Topics integral to this activity include the following:

- **Reporting relationships**. Simply, who reports to whom? Can they work together in a mutually and organizationally beneficial way?

- **Peer relationships**. Who relates to each other as peers, either within or across organizational units? Are they peers in terms of skills and stature?
- **Spans of control.** How large or small are the spans of control? Are they effective? Efficient? How do the spans of control interact with layers of the organization? Are there places where the desired span of control should be ignored for unique circumstances?
- **Layers.** How many layers are there? Is there a practical or philosophical limit? More layers create more bureaucracy, but might they also create more developmental opportunities and gradations? Would savings be achieved by eliminating a layer?
- **Communications.** Will the structure facilitate essential communications and hand-offs?

It is tempting to build the new organization around the skills and experiences of existing leaders, at both governance and management levels. A wiser approach is to focus on the needs of the new entity, use the strengths of current leaders, and fill out the structure with people from outside the current leadership team who have the skills needed to achieve desired results. While changing key individuals is uncomfortable, it may be necessary to accomplish the goals set for the new organization.

The new structure will be profoundly influenced by the forces driving the merger. A merger of equals requires intense negotiation and a balancing of interests. An explicit takeover allows the controlling organization to place its leaders in major roles but should also enable talented staff to expand their responsibilities. The ability to identify staff members to retain in a takeover is critically important, although a challenging task. It is particularly critical to monitor employee and physician perspectives during these situations.

Often, the overriding organizational issue in a merger is who the new CEO will be and, if both existing CEOs wish to remain with the new organization, what their roles and relationship will be post-merger. Sometimes, the situation is resolved fairly early if one or both CEOs retire or if the deal involves the assimilation of a small organization into a large one. However, frequently, who will become the CEO of the new organization is unclear, and the fate of the deal rests, in part, on the adroitness of the leaders in addressing this issue.

These situations are best dealt with by a small group of leaders, including (and sometimes limited to) the board chairs. While the choice of the new CEO should be based largely on the needs of the new organization and the relative capabilities and skills of the candidates, this is not always the case. Political and other considerations, as with other aspects of merger planning, will play a role here, too. Nonetheless, it is important to resolve this situation early in the discussion because, otherwise, the uncertainties of the situation are liable to disrupt the deal later in the process.

The first steps in creating the leadership structure were fairly easy for the boards of St. Elizabeth and St. Luke. The CEO of the larger organization, St. Elizabeth, would be the CEO of the new entity. His first action with the management structure was to assemble a senior management team for the system, including a new COO at each St. Luke hospital. Each senior executive was asked to develop an organizational chart for his or her division within three months of the merger. At a minimum, they had to identify

the management positions. The CEO and executive vice president then reviewed and modified these divisional charts to ensure essential working relationships throughout the new system.

Although the transition to the new organization has been very smooth, now a year into the merger (as of early 2010), each senior vice president has been asked again for his or her recommendations regarding leadership structure in the divisions. Why? In retrospect, the initial three-month evaluation was premature; not enough time had passed for leadership to be able to determine and resolve the practical issues that crop up in implementing any new organizational structure. After a year of merger experience and having had an opportunity to assess and compare the capabilities and competencies of managers across the organization, St. Elizabeth Healthcare leadership has more knowledge to address and enhance reporting relationships, peer relationships, span of control, organizational layers, and communications. This second wave of restructuring is also eliminating positions that are no longer needed.

At the time of the merger, the CEO made a public promise that no employee from either organization would lose his or her job as a result of the merger. This assurance stemmed from the growing community's need for additional healthcare services and the need for the newly merged organization to expand a number of corporate-type services. Leadership saw this public promise as a manageable commitment that would increase the rank-and-file employees' and community's support of the merger.

To fulfill this commitment, the organization reenergized a practice St. Elizabeth had used in the past—putting displaced employees in a temporary labor pool and paying them for up to 90 days while they, with substantial assistance from human resources, search for a job elsewhere in the organization. Despite the negative impact of the recent recession on local healthcare utilization, the new organization has successfully offered jobs to all displaced employees.

CONCLUSION

The organizational and operating structure of a newly created entity provides a foundation on which the opportunities that precipitated the merger are realized. When properly constructed, the new structure will encourage growth, promote efficient and effective governance and management, deal with the changing environment facing the new entity, assimilate disparate interests, and refocus everyone's energies on accomplishing the goals set for the organization.

CHAPTER 4 KEY TAKEAWAYS

- The most pressing concern in early merger discussions often is appointment of those who will be in charge and in control, but equally important is the design of the new organization. The way the new organization will be structured and operated will determine its eventual success or failure and touch the lives of everyone it employs.

- The choice between a joint operating agreement and an asset merger (as well as variants within these broad categories) may seem straightforward but often is not. Differences in culture and operating styles and a desire for some degree of autonomy may be barriers to full integration. A phased plan for full integration or a structure short of total assimilation may help balance competing concerns.

- When addressing the high-level relationships among business units, service lines, and other key corporate entities to create a new organizational and operational design, four variables must be considered: centralized versus decentralized, flat and broad versus narrow and deep, product and service compatibility, and the functions and value of each management layer.

- When the organization chart is developed with names or positions, reporting relationships, peer relationships, spans of control, layers, and communications must be examined to ensure pragmatic, day-to-day functionality.

- Newly merged organizations must focus on the needs of the new entity, use the strengths of current leaders, and look outside the current leadership team to fill out the structure with people who have the skills needed to achieve desired results.

Physician Impacts and Politics

KATHLEEN H. MCCARTHY

The goal or ideal outcome of physician strategy in a merger involving two or more hospitals or systems is to combine the talents, resources, and medical capabilities of the organizations' medical staffs to improve healthcare delivery in the communities served by the newly merged organization. Physician support tops the list of factors critical to a merger's success. Yet, physicians are often peripheral players in the merger transaction. Lack of attention to the possible effects of the transaction on physicians has the potential to derail the deal or prevent the merger from producing expected benefits.

This chapter identifies components of the physician practice and medical staff that should be evaluated when assessing the feasibility of a potential merger, frames the potential impacts mergers can have on physicians and offers strategies for addressing them, and outlines the benefits physicians might realize from the proposed transaction. While mergers and consolidations among physician groups are also occurring, this chapter addresses consolidation-related impacts on the members of the medical staffs of merging organizations.

PHYSICIAN AND MEDICAL STAFF COMPONENTS TO BE EVALUATED IN A MERGER TRANSACTION

The current medical staff profile, existing relationships between physicians and the hospital or system, and the physician culture each organization will bring to a merger transaction must be thoroughly and openly evaluated to anticipate and proactively address issues and opportunities. See Appendix 5.1 for key questions to consider in this evaluation.

Medical Staff Profile

The medical staff profile outlines the size and scale of the medical staffs at the merging organizations, identifies physician leaders and complementary clinical strengths, and probes perceived current and future physician needs by specialty. Some overlap of medical staff and familiarity with practice patterns and clinical capabilities among peers may help build a foundation of trust; however, if mutual dependence on a shared patient base without planned incremental growth exists, heightened competition among physicians may occur.

Degree of Physician Integration

Integration of physician practices, both practices joining together as well as practices merging with hospitals or systems, is increasing, and there is a growing differential between the ability of small practices versus large practices and hospitals/systems to address the following trends:

- Physician shortages are making recruiting more difficult and expensive.
- The current generation of physicians desires a work–life balance with predictable hours, call coverage, and time off.
- Private-practice economics are deteriorating as a result of static

or declining reimbursement, decreased contracting leverage caused by insurer consolidation, and increasing overhead costs.

The inability of physician practices and healthcare organizations to recruit an adequate number and mix of physicians has been a key driver of the current wave of provider consolidation. Organizations that have a practice management infrastructure and physician employment options have a competitive advantage because of their ability to more closely match practice opportunities with physician needs. Merging organizations with complementary physician networks have greater geographic coverage, greater potential to increase volume and market share, and a greater chance of achieving a more favorable negotiating position with managed care providers than they would have independently.

Breadth and Depth of Physician Alignment

The breadth and depth of options available to align physicians with a hospital or system are indicators of the strength of the organization's relationship with its medical staff and the level of physician engagement in the organization. Healthcare organizations with multiple strategies and options for physician alignment have greater flexibility to meet the needs of physicians in the potential partnering organization. Physicians who are closely aligned with a hospital or system are also less likely to defect during a merger but may feel at risk if they perceive that the proposed merger transaction would weaken the organization's financial performance or its market position.

Physician Culture

As discussed in Chapter 2, lack of cultural compatibility in organizations considering a merger is one of the most common obstacles to closing a deal and achieving the anticipated benefits of the merger. Identifying the physician culture each organization brings to the table and proactively managing potential pitfalls will reduce the likelihood that these differences will negatively affect the proposed partnership. For example, physicians in an academic environment tend to place priority on teaching and research activities, while community-based practitioners focus on patient care. Many employed physicians value economic security and a work–life balance over practice autonomy and independence, while the latter are paramount to private practitioners. The ability of these physician constituencies to coexist and work collaboratively toward a common goal is critical to the success of most merger transactions.

Potential Impacts of Mergers on Physicians

A merger could negatively affect the organizations' physician practices in three major ways:

- The physicians' professional income could decrease.
- The physicians could lose their independence and clinical autonomy.
- The physicians might have less control and influence at their hospital or system.

At the extreme, physicians may be concerned that the office space they own at one of the organizations may become a liability rather than an asset if the facility will close as a result of the merger or if clinical changes will be made post-merger.

The competitive environment and cultural differences that typically exist among physician segments (e.g., employed, private practice, faculty, hospital based) in a single organization become increasingly complex during a merger transaction. Drivers of these potential areas of conflict include the following:

- Consolidation of clinical programs at one of the sites increases the chance that existing referral and physician practice patterns will be disrupted and competition for patients among the merging organizations' physicians will intensify. Clinical departmental leadership positions could also be combined, which is of particular concern in academic settings.
- Restructuring of hospital-based physician contracts by the merging organizations could mean that physician groups in such services as anesthesiology, radiology, emergency medicine, and pathology are no longer the exclusive providers in their organization. Professional fee competition for interpretation of medical tests, medical and surgical consults, and inpatient visits may also result.
- Referrals that formerly went to independent private practitioners could be redirected to the employed physician network of one or both of the combining organizations. This threat often prompts valued independent physicians to defect from the current hospital

or system and sometimes from the service area, if local practice options are not readily available or are no longer attractive.

Each of the following case studies illustrates how a newly formed system addressed the impacts of the merger on its physicians.

THE NORTH SHORE HEALTH SYSTEM AND THE LONG ISLAND JEWISH MEDICAL CENTER

The North Shore Health System and Long Island Jewish Medical Center merged in 1997. The system has since grown to include 14 hospitals, ranks among the 20 largest healthcare networks in the country (on the basis of net patient revenue), and is among the nation's 100 most integrated healthcare networks, according to ratings by SDI, a healthcare data and consulting firm (North Shore-Long Island Jewish Health System 2010a, 2010b; SDI 2010).

The merging organizations' initial assumption was that merging the clinical programs at the two tertiary hospitals would create significant economies of scale and allow them to retain a full range of specialization and support functions. The anticipated consolidations that would have produced these economies met with strong resistance, and most were abandoned. Instead, principles of clinical integration were developed to guide collaborative programs that would help achieve specific goals, which included improved residency training, enhanced research opportunities, better quality of care, economies of scale, and improved clinical leadership. The principles of clinical integration were as follows (Cohen, Dowling, and Gallagher 2001):

- **Joint physician–hospital leadership**. Any proposal regarding clinical integration of a department, division, or program must include an analysis of the relationship between that department, division, or program and the hospital of which it is a part. This analysis must include input from senior hospital administrators regarding the pros and cons of integration.
- **Preservation of programs**. No program will be moved from one tertiary site to another without considering the interdependence of the program and related hospital departments at the location that would experience the program loss.
- **Optimizing quality, service, and growth at both hospitals**. The highest quality and service must be delivered to the communities

served while increasing market share of the clinical programs.

These guiding principles were applied when consolidation of the merging organizations' cardiac surgery programs presented a significant opportunity to reduce costs. The joint leadership group concluded that eliminating this service would negatively impact the character and mission of the newly merged organization and reduce referrals from the voluntary physician staff due to a perceived weakness in the reputation of the institution and its ability to draw patients from across the spectrum of diseases (Cohen, Dowling, and Gallagher 2001).

North Shore Health System and the Long Island Jewish Medical Center took a similar approach to integrating their faculty practice plans, which they saw as an important step toward clinical integration. A senior leadership team with administrative and clinical representatives from both organizations developed a set of guiding principles for the new practice plan. In addition to addressing research funding, levels of hospital support, and billing best practices through this process, the team developed multiple models of clinical departmental leadership.

By communicating a willingness to change the faculty practice plans despite the political, financial, and cultural challenges that the change would produce, the organizations demonstrated their commitment to the merger. The team's flexibility and patience in matching these models (e.g., one chairperson for each campus or both campuses, a co-chair/vice chair for each or both campuses, existing leaders versus new recruits) to the different circumstances of each department built trust within the organization and created an environment that encouraged and supported integration but never mandated it.

THE BRIGHAM AND WOMEN'S HOSPITAL AND FAULKNER HOSPITAL AFFILIATION   In 1998, Brigham and Women's Hospital and Faulkner Hospital developed a highly integrated affiliation under a common corporate parent, Brigham and Women's/Faulkner. Motivations for the affiliation were limited capacity at Brigham and Women's Hospital and excess capacity at Faulkner, and the need for Brigham and Women's Hospital to access lower-cost clinical space. The following points highlight the strategies the hospitals used to engage physicians and address potential concerns:

- The hospitals reached agreement on and clearly communicated each organization's role at the outset of the process. Community-level secondary care, including cases from Brigham and Women's Hospital, would be provided at Faulkner Hospital.

- A compelling case for growth was developed for both campuses that included a common goal for the physicians and administrative leaders of the combining organizations. By year three of the affiliation, Faulkner received over 5,000 incremental inpatients and outpatients combined as a result of shifting cases from Brigham and Women's to Faulkner. Instrumental to this shift of patients from Brigham and Women's to Faulkner was a contract with a large multispecialty group, Harvard Vanguard Medical Associates. Because the group received most of its reimbursement through full-risk capitation contracts, it had a financial incentive to extend its practice to a lower-cost community hospital setting. Implementation of the affiliation was continuously monitored to determine the impact of case shifting on quality, service, and finances at both hospitals.

- Faulkner's predominantly private-practice staff would retain its independence and standing within the medical staff. Maintaining the status quo in this regard was believed to be critically important to maintaining Faulkner's overall community hospital role and mission. These tenets became part of the affiliation agreement between the combining organizations.

- Multiple physician cultures were expected to coexist in the merged organization. The private practitioners at Faulkner coexisted with the physician organization at Brigham and Women's, which was a faculty/employed medical group, and with Harvard Vanguard Medical Associates. Several physician-led initiatives were developed that included all physician groups, including implementing care protocols and other quality initiatives across multiple care settings and locations. Chapter 6 of this book addresses the opportunities in this area in more depth.

The two hospitals also demonstrated a high level of sensitivity and communication about any integration initiative that could have been perceived as competition by any of the physician constituent groups. For example, the Brigham and Women's hospitalist program was extended to Faulkner to provide coverage for Brigham and Women's physicians at that location, but the hospitalist program was not mandated for private practitioners, many of whom continued to follow their own inpatients. In addition, primary care practices were shifted from Brigham and Women's to Faulkner, although they were predominantly mature practices with full patient caseloads that had been selected for relocation to minimize concerns about competition. Teaching programs were also consolidated, but vice chair roles were appointed in teaching departments at Brigham and Women's and Faulkner, creating a Brigham and Women's/Faulkner physician leadership team at each hospital to facilitate integration. Specialists also met monthly to discuss clinical service collaboration opportunities, clinical roles, coverage issues, and teaching responsibilities.

STRATEGIES FOR ADDRESSING POTENTIAL IMPACTS OF MERGERS ON PHYSICIANS

While these two case studies focus on post-merger integration, it is imperative to engage physicians in the premerger planning discussions about such topics as the selection of potential merger partners, the underlying rationale or justification for a proposed merger, and the perceived impacts and benefits of a potential merger on physicians. Physician input can be solicited through various means, including interviews, focus groups, task forces, and surveys. The process should be tailored to fit the cultures of the merging organizations. Multiple methods are often used; however, the methods for gathering input are less important than the quality of the communications, which should be meaningful to physicians and foster a sense of identity and ownership in the merger process.

The next step is to develop strategies for addressing physician concerns about the potential merger. Inclusion of the following "six Cs" is essential:

- **Clarity** about the proposed rationale for the merger transaction, including the potential impacts and benefits of the merger on physicians and the process/forum for clinical and financial decision making during the merger process

- **Communication** with physician constituencies initially and throughout the merger process
- **Compromise, creativity, and patience** among governance and administrative and physician leaders of the merging organizations
- **Culture**, including respect for the history, mission, and motivations of the combining organizations and their respective physician cultures
- **Common ground** between physicians and organizations in the merger process; physician engagement in quality initiatives and the development of coordinated programs of care
- **Control** and influence of physicians—discussion with physicians about their scope of control and evaluation of any changes that will result from the merger

CONCLUSION

Organizations that navigate successfully through the economic and political impacts that mergers have on physicians may realize a number of benefits:

- More opportunities for physicians to advance clinical program and professional development; increased ability to recruit and retain high-quality physicians
- Improved financial performance from top-line revenue growth and economies as a result of more scale, a stronger market position, and greater negotiating power with managed care companies
- Increased access to the latest technology, consulting services, and continuing medical education
- Expanded forum and opportunities for development and exchange of best practices
- Expanded academic affiliation
- Larger base of patient referrals, which enhances the training experiences of medical students, residents, and fellows and provides more candidates for research trials and development of clinical protocols

To achieve these benefits, the merger process must provide multiple opportunities for physician input and participation to ensure that their concerns are heard and their recommendations are vetted and implemented when feasible. Failure to manage these activities with sensitivity and care during the merger process could mean that the greatly anticipated benefits of the merger never come to fruition.

CHAPTER 5 KEY TAKEAWAYS

- Physician support is critical to the success of a merger; failure to involve physicians early and often in merger planning can derail a deal and prevent realization of expected merger benefits.
- A medical staff profile from each organization participating in the merger or acquisition must be thoroughly and openly evaluated; the profile should include an assessment of the degree of physician integration, the breadth and depth of physician alignment, physician culture, and potential impacts of the merger on physicians.
- Physician input should be sought on selection of potential merger partners, the underlying rationale for the proposed transaction, and the perceived impacts and benefits of the merger on physicians.
- The method for gathering input is less important than the quality of communications with physicians, which must be meaningful and foster a sense of identity and ownership in the merger process.

- The six Cs should be considered when addressing physician concerns: clarity; communication; compromise, creativity, and patience; culture; common ground; and control.

APPENDIX 5.1

Physician and Medical Staff Components to Be Evaluated in Merger Transactions: Key Questions to Consider

MEDICAL STAFF PROFILE
- How many physicians are there in each organization? What percentage of the medical staff provides primary care versus specialty care? What is their average age?
- What is the physician mix in terms of reputation, skills, and specialties? Are there physician champions who lead programs of distinction or centers of excellence?
- Where do the organizations' medical staffs overlap? Where are they complementary?

DEGREE OF PHYSICIAN INTEGRATION
- What percentage of the medical staff is employed versus in private

practice? How has this ratio been changing over the past few years?

- How large are the employed physician groups, and where are they located in the market to be served?
- What practice management infrastructure do the organizations have in place to support both employed and private-practice physicians?
- How many private-practice physician groups exist in the market, and what hospital/health system alliances have the groups developed?

BREADTH AND DEPTH OF PHYSICIAN–HOSPITAL/HEALTH SYSTEM ALIGNMENT

- What options do physicians have for alignment with the hospital or health system?

- What degree of alignment do these options achieve?
- What is the relationship between physicians and hospital/health system administration?
- How many and what type of physician leadership roles exist in each organization?

PHYSICIAN CULTURE

- What is the academic (teaching and research) presence in each organization?
- What degree of collegiality exists among the medical staff members?
  - Among primary care and specialty physicians?
  - Among employed and private-practice physicians?
  - Among academic and community-based physicians?

CHAPTER 6

Quality/Clinical Impacts

SUZANNE BORGOS

Quality improvement and clinical program development are often underlying rationales for mergers, yet such initiatives are typically the last to be instituted. They usually require a significant investment of time and resources, and results can take years to materialize. Achievement of quality and clinical goals is a challenge for healthcare organizations because they rely heavily on physician champions and involve controversial and politically charged decisions. Selection of clinical leaders and prioritization of clinical program development in the post-merger environment are even greater challenges.

This chapter outlines the components that potential partners should evaluate to determine the quality and clinical impact of a merger and set realistic expectations about the tasks ahead of them.

COMPONENTS OF A PREMERGER QUALITY ASSESSMENT

As pay-for-performance programs become more prevalent and have a greater impact on payment rates, healthcare is under increasing pressure to demonstrate excellent quality outcomes. Superior customer service and access to care are essential for organizations competing for referrals in a consumer-driven market. Consequently, most boards and senior leadership teams will continue to accept—if not expect—quality improvement as a justification for merger. The following actions can help organizations assess the degree to which quality of care can be improved through a proposed merger.

1. *Dedicate work groups to the premerger quality assessment.*

   Each entity should form a team of clinicians and quality leaders to review care delivery at each site. The teams should first identify relevant outcome and efficiency measures currently tracked across sites. Examples of such measures include the following:
   - **Centers for Medicare & Medicaid Services (CMS) Core Measures**: Process of care outcome measures for surgery, heart attack, pneumonia, and heart failure, available at www.hospitalcompare.hhs.gov
   - **National Patient Safety Goals**: Goals addressing such topics as patient identification, medication safety, and wrong-site surgery in ambulatory and inpatient settings, published annually by The Joint Commission (www.jointcommission.org)
   - **Patient satisfaction results**: Comparison of patient satisfaction survey results (e.g., Press Ganey, Hospital Consumer Assessment of Healthcare Providers and Systems [HCAHPS]) (HCAHPS data are available at www.hospitalcompare.hhs.gov.)
   - **Length of stay**: Evaluation of length of stay for high-volume discharges at each entity to measure efficiency and determine whether patient throughput can be improved

2. *Compare the structures, processes, outcomes, volumes, and efficiency measures of each entity involved in the merger against a national/regional benchmark.*

   As the teams analyze these measures, they should consider the following questions:

- Are there areas in which one significantly outperforms another?
- Do all entities perform exceedingly well, or could some locations benefit from sharing best practices?
- Is length of stay for high-volume discharges significantly different among the locations? If so, could adoption of best practices improve the patient throughput at the locations with longer lengths of stay?

Exhibit 6.1 provides examples of quality comparisons and identifies corresponding opportunities for each assessment.

3. *Identify action items for each site that could yield improvements in the quality of care delivery.*

    Potential action items should be developed on the basis of the opportunities identified in the comparison grid. Initial action items should involve clinical areas with high discharge or procedural volumes. Organizations often find it beneficial to concentrate on improving the care delivered to a targeted patient population. This task can be achieved through development of standardized clinical pathways and doctor's orders or

through establishment of disease-specific quality and patient safety committees.

Spectrum Health

In September 1997, Butterworth Health System and Blodgett Memorial Medical Center merged to operate jointly as Spectrum Health in Grand Rapids, Michigan. Formerly fierce competitors, these organizations combined their clinical pathway programs shortly after the merger to improve quality of care and encourage collaboration among multidisciplinary clinical teams (Schriefer et al. 2000).

Guided by the following steps, Spectrum Health was able to successfully consolidate clinical pathways across sites and gain the trust of both organizations' clinicians and senior leaders.

1. Conducted an inventory of previous clinical pathway efforts
2. Planned for an ideal program by incorporating best pathway practices from each of the sites
3. Brought staff together early in the merger process; encouraged open communication
4. Decided on a common clinical pathway format
5. Standardized the clinical pathway development and revision process

Quality Comparison	Opportunity
Hospital A scores better than Hospital B on most CMS core measures.	Hospital B could benefit from adopting Hospital A's clinical pathways in such areas as heart attack, heart failure, and pneumonia.
Hospital B has a better medication reconciliation compliance rate than Hospital A.	Hospital A could benefit from adopting Hospital B's (best) practices for medication reconciliation.
On average, Hospital A and Hospital B score at or above the Press Ganey 90th percentile in patient satisfaction.	Strong patient satisfaction is a point of synergy for these providers.

6. Standardized a clinical pathway reporting tool
7. Created a clinical pathway manual
8. Implemented a clinical pathway education plan for appropriate staff
9. Presented the clinical pathway program to physicians, nurses, and key administrative staff
10. Appointed an advisory group to direct the clinical pathway program going forward (Schriefer et al. 2000)

Communication and executive support were critical success factors in this initiative. Throughout the process, senior leaders allocated a significant amount of staff time and resources. From day one they encouraged open communication and transparency among stakeholders.

COMPONENTS OF A PREMERGER CLINICAL ASSESSMENT

Healthcare organizations have struggled to realize clinical benefits in a post-merger environment because initiatives such as program development, service line integration, and physician recruitment are typically met with skepticism and resistance. Clinical leaders at each site are fearful that their programs will be eliminated if services are fully integrated, and physicians are initially reluctant to work with new partners to develop joint programs. Furthermore, senior administrators often have difficulty selecting individuals to direct clinical initiatives; as a result, these decisions may be delayed for months or even years.

All too often, initiatives are implemented on the basis of unrealistic clinical integration goals. Entities that try to force programs together early on in a relationship can create a contentious work environment. By conducting the premerger clinical assessment outlined in the following list and communicating the results, potential partners ensure that all parties enter the transaction with the same expectations.

1. *Dedicate work groups to the premerger clinical assessment and charge them with identifying clinical synergies, complementarities, and redundancies.*
   - **Areas of potential clinical synergy**: When the strengths of one organization are combined with the strengths of another, the resulting combination/

collaboration is far stronger than each organization was on its own.
   - **Areas of potential clinical complementarity**: Typically, one organization has clinical strengths or capabilities that the other does not have; these strengths/capabilities can be extended to the other organization.
   - **Areas of clinical redundancy**: Duplicate clinical areas need to be evaluated to determine whether the redundancies are necessary.

Exhibit 6.2 provides a few examples of clinical synergies, complementarities, and redundancies that a premerger clinical assessment could identify.

2. *Evaluate the potential for service development and revenue enhancement for each service line by developing conservative, moderate, and aggressive future market growth and share scenarios.*
   - The evaluation should include calculations of the target market area(s) and share, estimated incremental cases, and estimated incremental contribution margin for each service

EXHIBIT 6.2: Examples of Clinical Synergies, Complementarities, and Redundancies

Synergies	Complementarities	Redundancies
■ A larger patient base will support development of a family practice residency program.	■ **Neurosciences:** Hospital A's neuro-interventional services and Hospital B's stroke center	■ Clinical laboratory ■ Diagnostic testing ■ Angiography suites ■ Pediatric inpatient units
■ Greater scale will facilitate physician recruitment.	■ **Long-term care:** Hospital A's acute care for the elderly unit and Hospital B's long-term care program	
■ High patient satisfaction at both sites will give the newly formed system a competitive advantage.	■ **Cardiovascular:** Hospital A's cardiac surgery program and Hospital B's outpatient cardiac rehabilitation services	

line and market share scenario. Often, a common objective is to reduce outmigration of more complex cases to other providers.

3. *On the basis of the analysis completed in steps 1 and 2, identify clinical areas that have the greatest potential for growth and joint program development.*

4. *Discuss the service redundancies identified in step 1, and determine* *how they may best be addressed in the post-merger environment.*

NewYork-Presbyterian Hospital

In January 1998, two large academic medical centers in New York City—New York Hospital and Presbyterian Hospital—merged to form NewYork-Presbyterian Hospital. The merger was largely justified by potential improvements in clinical quality and financial savings. After attempting to develop one set of medical bylaws and appoint clinical directors, senior administration realized that clinical integration could not be forced. Each center feared that integration efforts would result in favoritism of one hospital over the other and would weaken the programs and identity of both facilities. Thus, New York-Presbyterian instituted service lines to align the two clinical cultures and realize the benefits of integration without forcing the consolidation (Corwin et al. 2003).

Senior management developed four principles and required all service lines to adhere to them:

1. **Flexible**: Service lines do not have to use the same organizational model and will not be used to force consolidation or integration of departments.
2. **Inclusive**: The governance structure involves as many relevant individuals as possible.
3. **Physician-led**: Physicians determine the leaders of each service line and may designate multiple leaders.
4. **Transparent**: Data are shared among the hospitals, physicians, and affiliated medical schools for strategic planning, business planning, and performance tracking.

Senior management demonstrated their support for service line development by giving capital investment priority to service line projects. Their actions incentivized physicians to work together and establish common service line goals and objectives. Under this capital prioritization process, service line leaders had to commit to specific quality and medical management improvements. They were also required to work with administration to enhance customer service and increase revenue for the service line. If a service line met these criteria, it would receive capital investment priority (Corwin et al. 2003).

Since their inception in 1999, New York-Presbyterian Hospital's service lines have enjoyed tremendous success. By 2003, they accounted for 60 percent of discharges and 70 percent of revenues. Furthermore, service lines played a pivotal role in

- increasing discharges by more than 16 percent (86,000 before the merger to over 100,000 in 2002),
- decreasing length of stay by 10 percent (7.5 days in 1998 to 6.8 days in 2002),

- decreasing costs per discharge, and
- increasing service line market share in the New York metropolitan area (Corwin et al. 2003).

POTENTIAL BARRIERS TO IMPLEMENTING QUALITY AND CLINICAL INITIATIVES IN A POST-MERGER ENVIRONMENT

The final component of any pre-merger assessment is an evaluation of barriers that organizations may encounter when trying to implement post-merger initiatives. Here are a few examples of frequently encountered obstacles that may thwart or stall quality and clinical initiatives:

- **Organizational infrastructure and culture**. Quality and clinical program development initiatives in a post-merger environment often require former competitors to work together to achieve common goals. The infrastructure and culture of each organization will influence the ease with which they implement major initiatives. Organizations can evaluate this "ease of implementation" factor by answering the following questions:

- Do the senior leaders at each site support quality and clinical initiatives?
- Are there strong clinical and quality leaders at each site who are committed to collaboration, building trust, improving quality, and program development?
- Is there relevant multidisciplinary representation on existing quality and clinical committees (e.g., physicians, nurses, management, allied health)?
- Do the organizations have common service line and quality goals?
- Are individuals currently held accountable for quality improvement and service development at each entity?
- Are transparent and reliable quality/clinical data available?
- Is the opportunity for improvement significant, and is the improvement achievable?

- **Change is difficult**. Many people, especially those who have been in their profession or position for several years, become set in their ways and fearful of change. Clinicians typically show a degree of resistance to initiatives that will change the way they treat patients.

Therefore, end users should be involved in the premerger assessment and continually engaged as the merger proceeds.

- **Territorial instincts**. Clinicians naturally assume that a merger will consolidate existing programs and services and eliminate some or all of what was formerly "theirs." In the early stages of a merger, some individuals exhibit territorial behaviors to protect their turf. By developing trust among one another, administrative and clinical leaders can alleviate these tendencies and create a collaborative environment.
- **Different information systems**. Most post-merger initiatives, especially ones that involve inputting and evaluating data across entities, are difficult to implement when the merging organizations use different information systems. This obstacle can be fully evaluated during the premerger assessment.

CONCLUSION

Although potential clinical and quality benefits are not as easy to quantify as potential financial benefits, it is imperative that organizations establish multidisciplinary teams to identify what is feasible and achievable. The processes outlined in this chapter are intended to engage quality and clinical leaders in the premerger assessment phase and establish reasonable goals for each area in a post-merger environment. These early discussions should identify the challenges that lie ahead and shed light on the complexity of quality and clinical initiatives so that a full appreciation of implementation challenges is factored into post-merger planning. Mergers have enormous potential to positively affect quality improvement and clinical program development, but change will not occur overnight. Partners that understand the gradual nature of improvement will develop realistic expectations and reap greater rewards in the long run.

CHAPTER 6 KEY TAKEAWAYS

- Quality improvement and clinical program development are typically the last merger initiatives to be implemented; they require substantial investments of time and resources, rely on physician champions, involve politically charged decisions, and may take years to materialize.

- A premerger quality assessment should be conducted to determine the potential impact of a merger on quality of care and help both organizations reach a realistic understanding of the benefits and challenges that may result from the merger.

- A premerger clinical assessment may help the merging organizations prevent resistance from clinical leaders and others who are fearful that their program will be eliminated or scaled back as decisions are made about post-merger program development, service line integration, and physician recruitment.

- Barriers, such as organizational infrastructure, culture, difficulties embracing change, territorial instincts, and incompatible information systems may thwart or stall implementation of quality and clinical initiatives. Proactively identifying and managing these barriers in the premerger stages of planning may help neutralize their impact post-merger.

Financial Benefits

ROBERT F. HILL, JR.

Organizations can realize substantial financial benefits as a result of merger or acquisition, and the potential for financial benefits will always be a major decision-making factor in the planning process. Premerger/acquisition planning usually identifies operating cost savings, capital cost avoidance, and revenue enhancement as possible financial benefits. Organizations must make careful and conservative projections of these benefits for at least the first three years of operations, consider how they might be achieved, and forecast expenses they might incur as a result of a merger or acquisition. This chapter is a guide to assessing the financial benefits and costs of a merger or an acquisition.

PROJECTING THE FINANCIAL BENEFITS OF A MERGER/ACQUISITION

The following questions are points to consider when forecasting the financial benefits of a proposed merger or acquisition:

- What functions can or should be consolidated or centralized?
- What integration and synergistic opportunities exist?
- How can the performance of one or both organizations be improved?
- Where would standardization/ uniformity yield financial benefits?
  - Adoption of industry best practices?
  - Economies of scale?
  - Service development between the two organizations?
  - Other improvement opportunities?
- What are each organization's strengths and deficiencies by service and function?
  - How can those strengths be incorporated in/shared with/transferred to the other organization?
- What resources are required and what are the projected costs to plan for and implement the merger or acquisition (e.g., technology, people, capital)?
- What obstacles or constraints may affect the transaction, and how can they be resolved?
- What are the implications of all the previous on the relationships that all organizations involved in the potential merger have with physicians, clinical quality, staff/ employees, and the community?

Data from both organizations that typically are collected and reviewed to answer these questions are listed in Exhibit 7.1.

EXPENSE REDUCTION OPPORTUNITIES

Expense reductions should be anticipated in every merger or acquisition. Healthcare mergers or acquisitions typically yield expense reductions ranging from 2 to 10 percent annually (as a percentage of the organizations' combined total expenses). Staff reductions, which usually follow a merger or acquisition, account for some of these savings. In mergers of similar entities in the same market, these reductions may be substantial, while mergers between

EXHIBIT 7.1: Data Reviewed in Merger/Acquisition Planning Process

- Audited financial statements for the past three years

- Detailed internal financial and operating statements for the current year to date and the past two to three years

- Volumes and net revenue by major payer group/category for inpatient, outpatient, and emergency services

- Capital expenditure budgets for the current year and the next five to ten years (if available)

- Profit and loss analyses by service and payer, including net revenue and contribution margin for inpatient and outpatient volumes

- Pricing matrices (e.g., per diem and per unit of service)

- Bond statements or documents, including bond rating activities and actions over the past five years; audited financials for the past two to three years

- Performance metrics and monitoring reports used by management and/or the board in the following areas:

  - Cost monitoring, financial trends, and ratio analyses

  - Clinical benchmarking, service/quality benchmarking

  - External sources for comparative benchmarking

- Operating budgets for the current and upcoming fiscal year (if complete or in process)

- Long-term strategic plan, including financial plans or projections

- Any management action plans identifying management goals and objectives for the current or future years

organizations with little or no duplication of service areas may entail only modest reductions.

Healthcare mergers and acquisitions can typically achieve a 2 to 3 percent expense reduction in the areas noted in Exhibit 7.2. More aggressive expense reductions may be achieved with actions noted in Exhibit 7.3.

EXHIBIT 7.2: Opportunities for 2 to 3 Percent Annual Expense Reductions

- Reduction of senior-level management staff
- Consolidation of materials management functions
- Implementation of best practices for supply chain management
- Renegotiation of insurance contracts
- Streamlining of human resources operations and processes
- Centralization of professional/consulting contracts
- Centralization of support service contracts
- Consolidation of patient financial services
- Centralization of marketing/advertising contracts

Financial leaders generally work with external advisors to review organizations' staffing, operating, and other expense indicators. This evaluation includes comparison of full-time equivalent levels, salaries, benefits, and measures/costs per unit of production. From these data, the financial impact of anticipated future changes in such areas as staffing, service delivery, and program mix can be forecast. In the case of a merger, this process is typically a collaborative effort directed by senior leadership of both organizations. In the case of an acquisition, the ac-quiring organization typically performs these analyses.

INCREMENTAL EXPENSES INCURRED AS A RESULT OF MERGER/ACQUISITION

Organizations usually incur short-term incremental expenses in a merger/acquisition. These expenses generally include

- new organizational expenses (e.g., signage, stationary, advertising/ public relations),

EXHIBIT 7.3: Opportunities for Expense Reductions Greater than 3 Percent Annually

- More aggressive staff reductions
- Consolidation of select administrative/management departments and services
- Transition to lowest common salary and benefit ranges
- Widespread implementation of clinical best practices, especially clinical resource utilization management
- Consolidation of complex procedures/services at one site
- Closure of duplicate or low-volume services
- Closure or relocation of select services or sites/facilities
- Consolidation of physician groups with central management, scheduling, and so forth
- Debt refinancing/restructuring

- the cost of interfacing and integrating information systems,
- staff termination/severance expenses,
- unionization/labor relations expenses,
- legal and consulting fees, and
- vendor contract termination expenses.

These expenses can equate to millions of dollars and are an important consideration when informing boards of directors, management, and other stakeholders about the financial implications of the proposed merger or acquisition. In many situations, the incremental expenses offset almost all of the savings achieved in the first year of joint operation.

CAPITAL COST AVOIDANCE

The range of potential capital cost avoidance varies considerably from transaction to transaction, but the benefit can be substantial for healthcare organizations and the communities they serve. Organizations may be able to reduce capital investments in facilities, technology, and service development by

- reducing duplicative investments in clinical and support technology, equipment, and facilities;
- using compatible information technology systems; and
- relocating services from facilities that are near full occupancy to affiliated facilities that have underutilized capacity, thereby eliminating the need to add expensive equipment and expand/renovate at-capacity facilities.

Opportunities for capital cost avoidance can be identified by reviewing each organization's capital budgets (or plans) for the next five to ten years. A key variable in the determination of capital cost avoidance is the age of the organizations' equipment and facilities. The organizations' strategic plans or long-term goals can also be compared to see whether there are areas of overlap or opportunities to amalgamate priorities. One recent planning study involving a potential merger between two large health systems in the Midwest conservatively projected that the two parties could reduce capital expenditures by more than $200 million over the next ten years. The capital cost avoidance process also must take into consideration each organization's potential need for a capital infusion that it would be unable to raise on its own.

REVENUE INCREASES

Increased revenue is often the most significant financial benefit organizations can realize through a merger or an acquisition. Initiatives expected to drive up revenue include joint service development, service expansion and enhancement, program extension from one organization to the other, and improved reimbursement rates from third-party payers. Larger patient volume may also ease difficulties with recruitment of specialists and create opportunities to enhance programs that could reduce outmigration.

Inpatient revenue projections are based on expected number of patient days/admissions and expected revenue per patient day/admission for each payer class (e.g., Medicaid, Medicare, commercial, managed care). Outpatient revenue projections are based on expected outpatient visits/procedures and expected revenue per visit/procedure for each payer class.

Joint Service Development and Service Expansion and Enhancement

Service development usually involves

- identifying gaps in the continuum of services and prioritizing potential initiatives to fill these gaps,
- forecasting population-based demand and preliminary market share targets for candidate programs,
- analyzing geographic position in relation to target markets,
- recommending a limited number of programs for collaborative development and specific expected benefits,
- preparing a business case that includes a financial forecast, and
- identifying and addressing potential roadblocks to service development.

Program Extension

Merged organizations may also extend select services or product lines from one organization to the other when one organization possesses particular strengths or an outstanding reputation. Extending certain

services may enhance quality and increase volume and revenue.

Improved Payment Rates

Merged organizations may be able to contract for improved reimbursement rates from third-party payers. They may not be able to enjoy this benefit immediately after a merger or an acquisition because existing contracts may be in place for a specified period; however, upon renewal or renegotiation of the contracts, one or both organizations are often able to secure increases of 5 to 20 percent. While estimates of improved payment rates may be considered in merger planning, this subject should be approached carefully and cautiously, and the advice/guidance of legal counsel should be sought to avoid even the appearance of anti-competitive behavior. Exhibit 7.4 shows the range of projected expense reduction, capital cost avoidance, and revenue enhancement targeted for proposed mergers/acquisitions.

CASH FLOW IMPROVEMENTS

In addition to the cash flow effects of the areas discussed in this chapter (i.e., expense reductions,

Expense Reduction Range (Annually)	Capital Cost Avoidance Range (Onetime)	Revenue Enhancement Range (Annually)	Size of Combined Organizations (Total Expenses)
Central Pennsylvania Merger Between Two Small Health Systems[1]			
$4 million–$7 million	<$10 million	$5 million–$10 million	$560 million
Southwest Ohio Merger Between Two Large Health Systems			
$28 million–$56 million	$130 million–$170 million	$50 million–$75 million	$1.9 billion
Eastern Wisconsin Merger Between Two Large Health Systems			
$12 million–$25 million	$100 million–$390 million	N/A	$1.25 billion
New York State Merger Between Two Small Urban Hospitals			
$8 million–$13 million	N/A	$1 million–$2 million	$300 million

(1) Expense reduction and capital cost avoidance were projected to be minimal primarily because the flagship hospitals of the systems are located approximately 60 miles apart.

incremental expenses, capital cost avoidance, and revenue increases), merged organizations may also benefit from onetime cash flow improvements, such as the cash flow generated as a result of combining patient financial services and implementing best practices, which should reduce days in receivables. In addition, merged organizations may have more debt capacity and improved borrowing power.

PROJECTED PERFORMANCE

Financial projections are made by layering the potential impact of changes in expenses and revenue onto baseline projections of operating performance for each organization. Layering also enables projection of a broader set of financial performance indicators, including cash flow (sources and uses), total margin, fund balances, long-term debt, and return on assets. The financial planning model should include year-by-year projections for each of these indicators.

After the baseline and future financial performance have been projected, the projections should be tested in several possible future scenarios using different assumptions about market conditions, rate of program and market share growth, reimbursement trends, and operating models.

CONCLUSION

Financial benefits that may be realized from a merger or acquisition will always be a major consideration during the planning process. The effort to project these benefits should be thorough and meticulous; however, regardless of their magnitude, financial benefits should be a secondary consideration to other merger/affiliation decision-making criteria, such as fit with mission, vision, and values; alignment of strategic priorities; and cultural compatibility. If the entities involved in the proposed transaction are misaligned in any of these ways, their potential for achieving financial benefits will be diminished or eradicated entirely.

CHAPTER 7 KEY TAKEAWAYS

- Substantial financial benefits can be realized after a merger or acquisition, but careful and conservative projections must be developed, taking into account that incremental expense increases may offset savings in the early stages of the merger or acquisition.
- When projecting potential benefits, organizations should consider functions that could be consolidated or centralized, synergistic opportunities, standardization that could yield savings, organizational strengths and whether

they could be shared or transferred, resource requirements of the transaction, and relationships with physicians, clinicians, staff, and the community.

■ Healthcare mergers and acquisitions can typically yield annual expense reductions in the 2 to 10 percent range.

■ Increased revenue is often the most significant financial benefit that can be realized from a merger or an acquisition. Joint service development, service expansion or enhancement, and program extension from one organization to the other may yield incremental revenue.

CHAPTER 8

Other Issues and Concerns

ALAN ZUCKERMAN

Every acquisition or merger is unique and dynamic, with new issues emerging during premerger planning and in the years following completion of the transaction. The preceding chapters addressed the most common issues and concerns that surface in the initial stages of planning for mergers and acquisitions. This chapter identifies and describes additional challenges frequently encountered in merger or acquisition planning (see Exhibit 8.1).

HUMAN RESOURCE ISSUES AND CONCERNS

Significant human resource issues affect almost all mergers and acquisitions. Many of the subjects addressed in preceding chapters have

> **EXHIBIT 8.1: Secondary/Tertiary Merger and Acquisition Planning Issues and Concerns**

- Human resources
  - Staff reductions
  - Unions
  - Pensions
  - Benefits
  - Recruitment and retention
- Legal/regulatory
  - Antitrust
  - State attorney general
  - Certificate of need
  - Government sponsorship
  - Fair market value
- Religious
  - Sponsorship
  - The Catholic Church's ethical and religious directives
  - Conversion/identification
- Commitments
  - Hospitals or other facilities
  - Services
  - Capital
- Tertiary issues/concerns
  - Leadership opposition
  - Price/financial terms
  - Community
  - Brand recognition/image
  - Town/gown
  - Communication/transparency
  - Information technology
  - Facilities

implications for human resources, most notably culture, organization and operations, medical staff, and finance. Human resource issues are secondary only in the sense that they are not threshold concerns. In most instances, general agreement on the issues and concerns addressed in the first seven chapters of this book and an approach to managing them is needed before the more detailed and narrow human resource issues and concerns need to be confronted.

Staff Reductions

As discussed in Chapter 7, the potential for cost savings is usually a major impetus for pursuing a merger or acquisition. As a result, nearly all mergers and acquisitions involve some degree of staff reduction. In mergers of like entities in the same market, these reductions may be large, while an acquisition of an organization outside of the home entity's market may entail only modest reductions.

At this stage, the particulars of the reductions are not usually defined. Instead, the focus is on communications so that valuable staff are not lost and operations are not disrupted. Merger-related communications should be honest and reassuring but not misleading. Healthcare organizations have historically undercommunicated with their employees during merger planning. Instead, a concerted effort to be direct and forthright should be made.

Unions
When one organization has unions and the other does not, the spread of unions into the nonunionized organization becomes a concern. Highly qualified experts should be consulted about this specialized and technical area early on in the merger planning process to maximize the chance for a successful outcome.

Pensions
Merger or acquisition may lead to termination of one or more pension plans, or the new organization may absorb them in some form. Such changes involve myriad legal and financial issues (and require associated expertise) and have a significant impact on affected employees.

Benefits
Adjustment of benefits, either to make benefits uniform for all employees of the new organization or to achieve cost-reduction targets, is a common feature of mergers and acquisitions. Revision of benefits is a technical domain and requires specialized expertise to avoid legal issues, maximize financial improvement for (or minimize financial impact on) the merged entity, and avoid negative staff impacts.

Recruitment and Retention
A growing area of opportunity in the larger organizations that result from mergers and acquisitions is enhanced ability to recruit and retain staff. Recruitment of specialized personnel in particular is increasingly carried out in regional, state, national, and, in some cases, international markets; organizational size and scale are needed to succeed at recruitment of physicians and clinicians who are in short supply. On the retention side, size and scale offer opportunities for

professional development, training, and career development not possible in a smaller organization.

LEGAL/REGULATORY ISSUES AND CONCERNS

Legal and regulatory[1] issues and concerns are also secondary in that the business purpose and parameters of the merger/acquisition need to be established before these issues come to the forefront. The adage "form follows function" applies here. Nonetheless, legal counsel should be retained either from the outset or, at the latest, once formulation of a letter of intent or memorandum of understanding to proceed begins.

Antitrust

Probably the most commonly encountered issue and concern in mergers and acquisitions is the potential to violate, or be subjected to the scrutiny of, federal antitrust enforcement. If the new combination of organizations leads to high market concentration[2] and power, a Hart-Scott-Rodino[3] filing and federal review may be necessary. Even if high market concentration and power do not appear to be characteristics of a merger, legal counsel can offer valuable advice about how the parties can avoid the appearance of anti-competitive behavior and minimize the likelihood of subsequent government scrutiny (see Exhibit 8.2).

State Attorney Generals

Some states have activist attorney generals, often empowered by state statutes, who scrutinize healthcare transactions. Typically, the impetus for these inquiries is either antitrust regulation or oversight of public charities. Regardless of their purpose, if the deal is in a state where the attorney general's office has been known to intervene in mergers and acquisitions or a new activist attorney general has taken office, be prepared for scrutiny. In such situations, it may be prudent to take proactive action and inform the attorney general's office early in a potential transaction to minimize adverse consequences.

Certificate of Need

In states where certificate-of-need regulations are still in effect, merger or acquisition transactions may create a reviewable situation. Here, too, consultation with the appropriate agency early on may expedite the review process and lead to a higher likelihood of a timely and favorable review and decision.

EXHIBIT 8.2: Antitrust Guidelines for Written and Oral Communications

Words, Phrases, and Conduct to Avoid	Reason to Avoid
Guilty Words "Destroy after reading," "no copies," "for your eyes only"	Cast suspicion on the activity
Power Words "Control," "dominate," "dominance," "dominant position"	Suggest abuse of power
Negotiating Power "Increased bargaining power," "dominant position," "leverage," "clout"	Suggest power to increase profits
Phrases Suggesting No Realistic Competitors "Only seller," "essential seller"	Suggest power to raise prices and no choice
Words of Destruction "Eliminate," "destroy," "obliterate," "annihilate"	Suggest an intent to destroy or injure
Words Defining Markets or Market Share "75% of the [Product X] market"	Make market sound too narrow from an antitrust perspective
Words Suggesting Agreement Rather than Competition "Collaborate," "collaboration," "gentlemen's agreement," "partnering"	May imply an unlawful conspiracy
Words Suggesting Elimination or End of Competition "Eliminate the competition," "no choice but to buy . . ."	Imply unreasonable restraint or an anticompetitive effect
Words of Exclusion or Boycott "Exclude," "avoid," "boycott," "united front"	Suggest an anticompetitive intent or effect
Words Suggesting Power to Raise Prices "Enhance the bottom line," "increase profits," "leverage"	Suggest an intent to raise prices

SOURCE: McDermott Will & Emery (2009).

Government Ownership of Provider

Many municipally sponsored health-care organizations (usually city- or county-owned) are looking to join larger delivery systems. Mergers involving such entities are more complicated and complex than those involving private parties. State and/or local knowledge and expertise (legal and financial) will be required to determine how such a deal would be best accomplished.

Fair Market Value

The financial terms of the merger/acquisition of a for-profit entity by a not-for-profit one must not overstate the fair market value of the assets acquired. This issue is especially prevalent in the acquisition of physician practices. Involvement of valuation specialists and legal advisers is critical to preventing this situation.

RELIGIOUS ISSUES AND CONCERNS

A number of technical issues and concerns emerge in mergers and acquisitions involving a church-owned entity. Like the preceding concerns, these issues need to be addressed by advisers with relevant experience and expertise.

Sponsorship

A deal involving a faith-based entity may be subject to the sponsor's approval in addition to that of the board and local authorities. Decisions requiring approval should be anticipated early in the merger process, and, if possible, approval should be sought in advance of merger finalization to expedite completion of the deal. Mergers involving transfer of control from a church sponsor to another organization may be subject to additional scrutiny by church authorities and/or require more (or more complex) approvals. For example, the Vatican must approve the transfer of Catholic Church–owned property to a non-Catholic organization.

The Catholic Church's Ethical and Religious Directives

In transactions with Catholic health-care organizations, the Church's ethical and religious directives (regarding family planning and services prohibited by the Church, such as termination of pregnancy) may exert considerable influence. These directives may be extended to an acquired organization. In cases where certain services are no longer provided in the community as a result of these directives, community opposition to a lack of choice may arise and create political complications. Each diocese applies these directives differently, so consultation with local (and possibly system) authorities is important.

Conversion/Identification

If the acquiring entity is faith based but the entity to be acquired is not, the acquirer may require the acquired entity to be operated as a faith-based organization, and vice versa. When an acquired faith-based entity becomes nonsectarian, it may insist on retaining some physical or other identifiers associated with its heritage. Conversion may also occur in mergers of faith-based and non-faith-based organizations. Addressing these issues in mergers is less straightforward than in an acquisition.

COMMITMENTS

When a not-for-profit organization acquires another not-for profit organization, money is not usually exchanged, but the entity to be acquired often seeks assurances and commitments up front about certain actions the acquiring entity will take post-acquisition. As noted earlier, these commitments may relate to governance, organizational form and

function, and staff retention, but they are just as likely to pertain to three other major concerns: facilities, services, and capital. Commitments in these three areas are also common in for-profit acquisitions of not-for-profits.

Hospitals or Other Facilities

Keeping a hospital and other important facilities open and in full service for a predetermined period is often a precondition in a merger or an acquisition. This condition is especially common in deals involving smaller or rural facilities. A five-year commitment is typically requested, but it may be as short as three years or as long as ten years.

Services

Similarly, the acquired organization may seek a commitment that some or all of its services not be terminated or reduced in scope for some specified period.

Capital

Many organizations seeking to be acquired are looking for a capital infusion into their organization that they are unable to raise on their own. Historically, requests have ranged from fairly modest capital commitments ($5 million to $10 million) to rebuilding a hospital entirely, which is not uncommon in for-profit acquisitions of rural not-for-profit hospitals or municipally owned facilities.

TERTIARY ISSUES AND CONCERNS

The issues and concerns discussed in the following paragraphs are generally less typical than those discussed thus far.

Price/Financial Terms

Transactions that involve not-for-profit entities only (including municipally owned organizations) generally do not involve an exchange of money. However, if the acquired entity has substantial reserves, there may be discussion about how they will be used. The handling of existing long-term debt may also be a point of discussion. In transactions involving for-profit organizations (and occasionally not-for-profits as well), valuation of assets to be acquired is critical and specialized valuation advisers are generally needed in the acquisition planning process.

Leadership Opposition

The assumption underlying the information in this chapter is that leadership of the acquired organization fully supports the transaction.

However, aspects of the deal are sometimes unappealing to certain constituents. A minority opposition group may emerge as the discussions ensue. Be prepared for some level of dissent in any transaction.

Community

The impact an acquisition will have on the acquired entity's community (or a merger's impact on multiple communities) should be addressed from the outset of the transaction. Political and substantive concerns, such as unease about reductions in service, staff layoffs, and impacts on the local economy, may arise, and a proactive plan to address these issues is necessary.

Brand Recognition/Image

Sometimes an acquired organization is looking for an identity makeover or at least a brand boost. No matter what the reputation of the acquiring entity is, such brand improvement or transfer will not occur automatically. Marketing/public relations investments and interventions will be required.

Town/Gown

In combinations involving university-affiliated and community-based organizations, academic/faculty culture and behaviors may clash with those of community-based organizations and voluntary physicians. These conflicts are among the most difficult issues to address and generally require a high degree of creativity, flexibility, and years of effort to successfully resolve.

Communications/Transparency

Mergers and acquisitions are disruptive endeavors. They change an organization's direction and affect the lives of people working in it. Whenever possible, open and ongoing communication about what is to come is critical. Once a potential merger or acquisition has become public, a communications plan should be implemented and revised as necessary as the deal proceeds to ensure affected constituencies are involved and aware, to the extent appropriate.

Information Technology

Because of the magnitude of current and future spending on IT, at a certain point in the planning process a focus on IT needs and integration potential is appropriate.

Facilities

Facility needs, capital requirements, and any significant changes to the use of involved facilities must be evaluated as planning proceeds.

CONCLUSION

Mergers and acquisitions are unique and present multifaceted challenges in premerger and post-merger phases. This book has catalogued and described primary issues and concerns, and this chapter has touched on the most common secondary and tertiary issues. I hope organizations in the beginning stages of merger or acquisition planning find this information useful; those still contemplating the idea now know what to anticipate if they decide to proceed.

NOTES

1. None of this content should be construed as legal advice.
2. Regulators use the Herfindahl-Hirschman Index to measure the size of firms in relation to the industry or market in which they operate and to determine their competition.
3. The Hart-Scott-Rodino Improvement Act of 1976 is a set of amendments to the antitrust laws of the United States. It requires that the Federal Trade Commission and U.S. Department of Justice be notified of potential mergers of a certain size. (The size criteria are adjusted over time.)

CHAPTER 8 KEY TAKEAWAYS

- Significant human resource issues emerge during mergers and acquisitions, particularly in the areas of culture, organization and operations, medical staff, and finance; detailed human resource issues cannot be addressed until general agreement on the merger or acquisition is reached and a clear approach to it is developed.

- Legal counsel should be retained by both parties at the outset of merger discussions or, at the latest, once a letter of intent or memorandum of understanding to proceed is under development.

- When church-owned entities are involved in a merger or acquisition, either as the acquirer or acquired organization, additional issues, such as sponsorship, ethical and religious directives, and conversions/identification may need to be addressed. Advisers with experience in these areas should be sought early in affiliation discussions.

- When not-for-profit healthcare organizations merge with one another, or a not-for-profit is acquired by a for-profit organization, assurances and commitments about certain actions may be requested. Concerns about facilities, services, and capital are most common, but concerns about governance, organization form and function, and staff retention may also arise.

- Other tertiary concerns, such as pricing and financial terms, opposition to the merger, community issues, university-affiliated versus community-based organizational priorities, effective communication, information technology, and facilities, may present additional challenges for merging organizations and should be managed proactively whenever possible.

References

Advocate Health Care. 2010. "Advocate Welcomes BroMenn into the System." [Online press release; retrieved 3/20/10.] www.advocatehealth.com/bromenn/body_noFAD.cfm?id = 130& action = detail&ref = 61.

———. 2009. "Illinois Health Board Approves Advocate Health Care, BroMenn Healthcare COE." [Online press release; retrieved 10/21/09.] www.advocatehealth.com/body.cfm?id = 12& action = detail&ref = 37.

Alltucker, K. 2008. "Banner Completes Acquisition of Sun Health." [Online article; retrieved 4/22/10.] www.azcentral.com/business/articles/2008/09/03/20080903biz-banner0903.html.

———. 2007. "Banner, Sun Health to Merge." [Online article; retrieved 11/30/09.] www.azcentral.com/arizonarepublic/local/articles/0922banner0922.html?&wired.

BroMenn Healthcare. 2008. "BroMenn in Talks to Partner with Advocate Health Care System." [Online press release; retrieved 10/21/09.] www.bromenn.org/News/bromenn-in-talks-to-partner-with-advocate-health-care.aspx.

Cohen, J. R., M. Dowling, and J. S. T. Gallagher. 2001. "The Trials, Tribulations, and Relative Success of the Ongoing Clinical Merger of Two Large Academic Hospital Systems." *Academic Medicine* 76 (7): 675–83.

Corwin, S., M. Reich Cooper, J. Leiman, D. Stein, H. Pardes, and M. Berman. 2003. "Model for a Merger: NewYork-Presbyterian's Use of Service Lines to Bring Two Academic Medical Centers Together." [Online article; retrieved 10/21/09.] http://journals.lww.com/academicmedicine/Fulltext/2003/11000/Model_for_a_Merger__NewYork_Presbyterian_s_Use_of.7.aspx#.

Gonzales, A. 2007. "Banner Health to Merge with Sun Health." [Online article; retrieved 10/11/09.] http://phoenix.bizjournals.com/phoenix/stories/2007/09/17/daily55.html.

Grand Rapids Press. 2009. "Spectrum Health, Area's Largest Physician Group MMPC in Merger Talks Again." [Online article; retrieved 10/11/09.] www.mlive.com/news/grand-rapids/index.ssf/2009/05/spectrum_health_areas_largest.html.

Lencioni, P. 2002. "Make Your Values Mean Something." *Harvard Business Review.* [Online article; retrieved 10/2/09.] http://harvardbusiness.org/product/make-your-values-mean-something/an/R0207J-PDF-ENG.

Steven H. Lipstein (CEO and president, BJC HealthCare), in discussion with Alan Zuckerman, December 1, 2009.

Mallon, W. T. 2003. "The Alchemists: A Case Study of a Failed Merger in Academic Medicine." *Academic Medicine* 78 (11): 1090–104.

North Shore-Long Island Jewish Health System. 2010a. "About Us: Facts and Statistics." [Online information; retrieved 6/23/10.] www.northshorelij.com/NSLIJ/Facts + and + Statistics + About + North + Shore-LIJ.

———. 2010b. "Hospitals and Centers: Member Hospitals." [Online information; retrieved 7/15/10.] www.northshorelij.com/NSLIJ/Member + Hospitals.

Sanford Health–MeritCare. 2009a. "Sanford and MeritCare Create a New Health System." [Online press release; retrieved 11/30/09.] www.sanfordmeritcare.com/sanford-and-meritcare-create-a-new-health-system.

———. 2009b. "Sanford and MeritCare Sign Letter of Intent to Create a New Health System." [Online press release; retrieved 10/11/09.] www.sanfordmeritcare.com/sanford-and-meritcare-sign-letter-of-intent.

Schriefer, J., J. Engelhard, L. DiCesare, M. Miller, and J. Schriefer. 2000. "Merging Clinical Pathway Programs as Part of Overall Health System Mergers: A Ten-Step Guide." *Journal on Quality Improvement* 29 (1): 29–38.

Schroder, G. 2008. "Merger Talks End for MMPC, Spectrum Health." [Online article; retrieved 10/11/09.] http://blog.mlive.com/grpress/2008/06/merger_talks_end_for_mmpc_spec.html.

SDI. 2010. "SDI Top 100 IHNs™—National." [Online information; retrieved 7/15/10.] www.sdihealth.com/IHN/SDI_2010_Top_100_IHN_National.pdf.

Spectrum Health. 2009. "mmpc to Integrate into Spectrum Health System." [Online press release; retrieved 10/11/09.] www.mmpc.com/spectrum_health_integration.

Suburban Hospital. 2009a. "Suburban Hospital Healthcare System to Join Johns Hopkins Medicine." [Online press release; retrieved 10/21/09.] www.suburbanhospital.org/news/PressReleaseDetails.aspx?prid = 67.

———. 2009b. "Suburban Hospital Healthcare System Joins Johns Hopkins Medicine." [Online press release; retrieved 10/21/09.] www.suburbanhospital.org/News/PressReleaseDetails.aspx?prid = 71.

UPMC. 2009a. "Our Mission, Vision, and Values." [Online information; retrieved 10/21/09.] www.upmc.com/aboutupmc/TheUPMCStory/governance/Pages/mission-vision-values.aspx.

———. 2009b. "The UPMC Story." [Online information; retrieved 10/21/09.] www.upmc.com/aboutupmc/TheUPMCStory/Pages/default.aspx.

———. 2009c. "UPMC Fast Facts." [Online information; retrieved 10/21/09.] www.upmc.com/aboutupmc/fast-facts/Pages/default.aspx.

Acknowledgments

They start with Pete. Our late colleague and friend Pete McGinn was the force behind the concept of a book on mergers and acquisitions for healthcare leaders. He did all the initial legwork, drafted the first sample chapter, and convinced us that rather than have one or two senior staff write the book, this publication would benefit from the insights of multiple contributing authors. Pete also helped the authors solidify their chapter outlines and helped them get started on the difficult task of writing their chapters. And then, unfortunately and prematurely, Pete passed away. This book is dedicated to him.

We benefited greatly from experiences in mergers and acquisitions consulting with our clients and from insights offered collectively in the field. Thanks especially to Joseph Gross of St. Elizabeth Healthcare, Steven Lipstein of BJC HealthCare, Scott Powder of Advocate Health Care, John Prout of TriHealth, and Michele Lawrence of University of Rochester Medical Center. Many others, too numerous to mention, helped along the way by sharing their experiences and those of their organizations.

As always, the Health Strategies & Solutions team did a marvelous job behind the scenes. Susan Arnold turned much of our inelegant writing into comprehensible and insightful prose. Kelly Raible helped with research and general all-purpose support. Others pitched in and provided important, focused assistance.

Finally, I want to thank the Health Strategies & Solutions consultants who "volunteered" to write the chapters of this book that Pete and I didn't author. In most instances, this work was their first contribution to a book and a significant step up from writing reports, articles, newsletters, and other shorter pieces. Congratulations to Suzanne Borgos, Maria Finarelli, Robert Hill, Kathleen McCarthy, Keith Pryor, Mike Walters, and Samuel Steinberg for a job well done!

Enjoy and good luck with your consolidation initiatives!

Alan M. Zuckerman, FACHE, FAAHC
Philadelphia, Pennsylvania
April 2010

About the Contributors

Suzanne Borgos is a manager with Health Strategies & Solutions, Inc. She has both clinical and strategic planning expertise, with particular emphasis on clinical integration and operational performance improvement. Prior to joining Health Strategies & Solutions, Suzanne held several administrative positions in the North Shore-LIJ Health System. Most recently, she was senior administrative director for neurosurgery, with responsibility for day-to-day operations, marketing, strategic planning, and programmatic growth.

Maria Finarelli is a principal with Health Strategies & Solutions, Inc., and has nearly 15 years of experience as a healthcare consultant. Maria manages the firm's complex planning engagements, including strategy development and demand forecasting projects. Her extensive skills in competitive positioning and developing market analyses and population-based demand forecasts have provided her clients with detailed, comprehensive data and recommendations on how to plan future programs and services.

Robert F. Hill, Jr., FACHE, is a principal with Health Strategies & Solutions, Inc., and has nearly 20 years of healthcare consulting experience. Robert directs Health Strategies & Solutions' financial planning and compliance practice, including the financial analyses associated with affiliation and partnership evaluations. Robert received the American College of Healthcare Executives' Service Award for his commitment and service to the healthcare management profession and the Early Career Award from the American College of Healthcare Executives' Southeastern Pennsylvania Regent in recognition of his efforts in advancing healthcare management excellence.

Kathleen H. McCarthy is vice president of Health Strategies & Solutions, Inc. With more than 20 years of experience in the healthcare industry as an executive and a consultant, Kathleen plays a key role in the firm's merger, acquisition, and affiliation client engagements, especially with regard to physician issues. Her ability to identify key strategic issues and build consensus on strategies for moving organizations forward has enabled providers to create vibrant strategic plans, grow volume and market share, develop thriving clinical programs, and build high medical staff alignment.

Peter V. McGinn, PhD, was a senior strategist with Health Strategies & Solutions, Inc., until his death in 2009. Peter was a highly regarded healthcare executive and consultant with over 25 years of experience in healthcare leadership. Peter held management positions in academic organizations, complex systems, and community healthcare, including serving as chief executive officer of United Health Services, a merged healthcare system in Binghamton, New York, and vice president for human resources at the Johns Hopkins Hospital and Health System in Baltimore. Peter was the author of *Leading Others, Managing Yourself* and *Partnership of Equals: Practical Strategies for Healthcare CEOs and Their Boards*, both published by Health Administration Press.

Keith T. Pryor is director of Health Strategies & Solutions' leadership advisory services practice, with expertise in change management, cultural alignment, strategy execution, specialized leadership coaching, and governing board effectiveness. Formerly a health system chief executive officer, Keith has served on the faculty of Cornell University's Sloan Program in Health Care Management; as principal with Diversified Search, Inc., a leading healthcare executive retained search firm; and as director, Key Executive Services, for Right Management Consultants, a highly regarded organizational consulting firm.

Samuel H. Steinberg, PhD, FACHE, has had a distinguished career in the healthcare field. He has held senior management positions, including chief executive officer, in five academic medical centers and has been a faculty member of five colleges and universities. Most recently, he has been serving as a consultant for a variety of healthcare organizations, including pediatric, specialty, community, and major teaching hospitals. He is the author of many articles and one book, *The Physician's Survival Guide to the Hospital*.

Michael J. Walters, PhD, is a senior strategist with Health Strategies & Solutions, Inc. Providers benefit from Michael's expertise in healthcare strategy and execution, merger and acquisition planning, and post-merger integration, which draws on 30 years of experience as a healthcare executive, consultant, and educator. Prior to joining Health Strategies & Solutions, Michael served as senior vice president, system development, at St. Elizabeth Medical Center in Edgewood, Kentucky, where he played a key role in facilitating post-merger activities and consolidating services.

About the Editor

Alan M. Zuckerman, FACHE, FAAHC, is president of Health Strategies & Solutions, Inc., and one of the nation's leading healthcare strategists. He has helped many top hospitals and health systems develop advanced competitive strategies and pursue affiliation activities. A healthcare management consultant for 35 years, Alan is the author of over 75 articles and five books, including *Healthcare Strategic Planning: Approaches for the 21st Century*, which won the 1999 American College of Healthcare Executives' James A. Hamilton Book of the Year Award.